Memories of Distant Places

Korea in the Vietnam War Era 1961-1965
A Memoir

A. L. Provost

MEMORIES OF DISTANT PLACES
Korea in the Vietnam War Era 1961-1965 A Memoir
Copyright © 2021 by A.L. Provost

All rights reserved. No part of this publication may be reproduced, distributed, or transmitted in any form or by any means, including photocopying, recording, or other electronic or mechanical methods, without the prior written permission of the publisher or author, except in the case of brief quotations embodied in critical reviews and certain other noncommercial uses permitted by copyright law.

Although every precaution has been taken to verify the accuracy of the information contained herein, the author and publisher assume no responsibility for any errors or omissions. No liability is assumed for damages that may result from the use of information contained within.

Library of Congress Control Number: 2021916071
ISBN-13:   Paperback: 978-1-64749-586-2
           ePub: 78-1-64749-587-9

Printed in the United States of America

GoTo Publish
GoToPublish LLC
1-888-337-1724
www.gotopublish.com
info@gotopublish.com

Contents

Prologue
Introduction

Chapter 1
The Improbable Adventure Begins 1

Chapter 2
I Enlist in the U.S. Army – The Adventure Begins 13

Chapter 3
A Most Fortuitous Conversation 21

Chapter 4
A Most Interesting Life Begins 31

Chapter 5
The Luckiest G.I. in Korea 37

Chapter 6
The Bridge that Wasn't There Or What Happened to My Bridge? 49

Chapter 7
The Korean Dictator's Press Conference My Frightening
Near-death Experience 59

Chapter 8
Confrontation Inside the Joint Security Area 65

Chapter 9
Return to Camp Page (The Honest John Rocket Revisited) 83

Chapter 10
The Drowned Communist Spy Inside
The Japanese Midget Submarine 91

Chapter 11
The Offer I Couldn't Refuse 111

Chapter 12
U.S. Army Intelligence Center Ft. Holabird, Maryland – 1964 131

Chapter 13
First Interrogation 139

Chapter 14
End of First Day at the 502 155

Chapter 15
    Interrogation Techniques 161
Chapter 16
    Incompatible Goals of Agents and Minders.. 167
Chapter 17
    My First Prisoner's Execution 173
Chapter 18
    Investigating the Communist Economy 181
Chapter 19
    My Second Prisoner: Fate of the Wounded Enemy Agent 187
Chapter 20
    My Third Prisoner: A Political Mystery Who Was James
    William Fulbright?... 195
Chapter 21
    Had I Bitten Off More Than I Could Chew? 203
Chapter 22
    My Fourth Prisoner: The Paratrooper The Nakasankanghaja Yundae
    (The Hidden Paratrooper Regiment) 211
Chapter 23
    Lone Agent – Three-man Team – Lone Agent....................................... 221
Chapter 24
    Those Insidious Stomache Pains Begin 231
Chapter 25
    I Receive a Friendly Warning 237
Chapter 26
    My Fifth Prisoner: A Change in Tactics? Family Members as
    Hostages: An Issue of Trust 241
Chapter 27
    My Sixth Prisoner: A Liar's Trip to Yongsan: The Polygraph................. 249

Epilogue

Praise for the Mystery Novels of A. L. Provost:

The Sharecropper's Daughter's Secret
...fascinating...attention grabbing...morally-compelling.
Writer's Digest

The Tangled Web
Congratulations on a great book that combines historic detail with suspense and superb characterization.
Writer's Digest

The Thirty-seventh Parallel
You did a good job building the suspense and drawing the reader into the plot.... I found myself reading quickly without realizing how much time was passing.
Writer's Digest

The Puppeteer
The murder plot that unravels in the novel is complex and well-developed.
Writer's Digest

Grand Deceptions
...deals with intricate plots that unfold over a relatively brief period of time.
Writer's Digest

The Bookmark Murders
...carefully constructed narrative travels at a good pace.
Writer's Digest

The Price of Greed
...writing is very meticulous and clear.
Writer's Digest

The Trust of Old Men
...it's clear that the plot of the book was well thought-out.
Writer's Digest

The Holstein Diamonds
...intelligent thriller with a compelling premise.
Writer's Digest

The Road to Dresden
...compelling and fascinating World War II thriller.
Writer's Digest

ALSO BY A. L. PROVOST

Reflections in an Orphan's Eye
A Decade at Oxford 1947-1957

The Puppeteer
The Tragedy of the Fifteen Days

Deception at Los Alamos
The Race for the Atomic Bomb 1940-1945

The Thirty-seventh Parallel
Planning the Second Korean War

The Tangled Web
Retaking the Nazi Diamonds

Grand Deceptions
The Plot to Kill FDR

The Bookmark Murders
Saving Emil Heider

The Price of Greed
The 1944 Camp Lejeune Payroll Heist

The Unwilling Spy
Testing the Atomic Bomb–1943

The Trust of Old Men
The Coastal Plain Conspiracy

The Sharecropper's Daughter's Secret
Finding Hedgeworth's Fortune

One Thief Too Many
Anatomy of a Bank Heist

A Gathering of Thieves
A German Immigrant's Tragedy

The Road to Dresden
Another Tangled Web-1942

The Holstein Diamonds
And the Cobbler's Rockery

Death is Waiting
Saving Mae Carter

Memories of Distant Places
Korea in the Vietnam War Era 1961-1965
A Memoir

Dedication

With the greatest respect and admiration, this memoir is dedicated to the American soldier, without whose sacrifices none of us would be free.

I'll Never Forget Sam Winfield

I was born on April 30, 1939, in Kinston, North Carolina, the sixth child and the fifth son of Nina Pearl and Benjamin Daniel Provost.

Exactly four months later, on August 30, 1939, young Samuel F. Winfield arrived at historic Oxford Orphanage (estab. 1872), located in the small town of Oxford, North Carolina, a couple of dozen miles due north of the tobacco town of Durham.

During World War II my dad worked for the federal government as a refrigeration engineering supervisor at the Cherry Point Marine Air Station on the east coast of North Carolina.

The war with Japan ended in August 1945, and my dad continued working at his engineering job at Cherry Point. On February 9, 1946 my dad died, leaving a widow and seven children for her to raise. Several months later my four older brothers, Bill, Kenny, Norwood and John, moved to Washington, D.C. to live with our relatives.

In August 1946 my only sister Eoline, two years older than I, was taken to Oxford Orphanage, and on February 15, 1947, at age 7, I followed my sister. Reluctantly.

The sprawling 400-acre orphanage campus and grounds, that included the farm and a 50-cow dairy, was home to a maximum of 346 students. If a boy was three years older than you, he was simply referred to as a "big boy."

We took our meals, "family-style," in two large dining rooms, and children of all ages mingled together as we awaited the bell that called us inside.

Everyone liked Sam "Greek" Winfield. He excelled in football and baseball as well as scholastics, and in 1947 he was mentioned on the all-North Carolina football team. He was no doubt the most popular student on campus.

Sam graduated high school in May 1948. After spending the fall 1948 semester at East Carolina Teachers College (E.C.T.C., now East Carolina University) in Greenville, located about an hour's drive north of Kinston, Sam enlisted in the U.S. Army. He quickly rose to the rank of corporal in a tank unit of the 25th Division, stationed with the U.S. Army's Occupation Forces in Japan.

On June 25, 1950 we read in the Durham *Morning Herald* and the Raleigh *News and Observer* that troops from a country named *North Korea*, known as the *communists*, had invaded a country named *South Korea*. Units of the 25th Division were rushed to South Korea to fight the invading communists, that we called the *gooks*.

Sam Winfield was killed in action in South Korea on August 12, 1950.

He was only 22 years old.

I cried when I heard the news.

What is a "communist," I wondered.

And where is this North Korea? It seemed so far away.

We children had a hard time coming to grips with the reason Americans like our friend Sam Winfield had to travel all the way around the world to fight and die for people who were not even American.

It all came together twelve years later, beginning in the early hours of January 2, 1962, when I and 999 other G.I.s stepped off a troopship in Inchon harbor onto South Korean soil. Events of the ensuing nearly four years (January 1962-November 1965) would provide some of the answers to these seminal and disturbing questions. However fifty-three years after leaving Korea for the last time (November 4, 1965) I fear that the questions may never be answered to my satisfaction.

My Reason for Writing This Memoir
A Snapshot in Time

North Korea and South Korea will be on the minds of world leaders until the United States ends Kim Jong Un's iron-fisted control of North Korea.

Memories of Distant Places presents an up close and personal account of the two Koreas during the four-year period January 1962-December 1965.

On May 15, 1961 General Park Chung Hee took control of the South Korean government in a lightning but bloodless coup. The following day, May 16, 1961, I graduated Berry College and six weeks later, on June 30, 1961, enlisted in the U.S. Army.

For fifteen months in 1962-1963 I roamed freely throughout South Korea as the sole feature writer and youngest reporter for the *Stars & Stripes* daily newspaper, writing about civilian and military life. I traveled alone in my own personal Jeep over dusty roads during dry weather and muddy roads during the rainy season, studying the Korean language every day. In addition I attended and reported in the *Stars & Stripes* on every Military Armistice Commission (MAC) meeting held in Panmunjom. During these exciting fifteen months never was the accuracy of my reporting questioned by Col. George Creel, my boss and the Eighth U.S. Army Information Officer, nor Sergeant Warren Kelsey, *Stars & Stripes* Bureau Chief.

After joining U.S. Army Intelligence in 1963, I attended the Defense Language Institute (DLI), where I studied Korean for 47 weeks, then studied Prisoner of War Interrogation for eight weeks at the U.S. Army Intelligence Center at Ft. Holabird in Baltimore. Then I returned to Korea where I interrogated North Korean espionage agents for sixteen months in 1964-1965, as the youngest prisoner interrogator.

I am certain that during this period I knew more about South Korea and North Korea than did any other American.

My Knowledge of The Two Koreas

My first-hand knowledge of *South Korea* is drawn from my first U.S. Army tour of duty encompassing my fifteen months as the only feature writer for the *Pacific Stars & Stripes* daily newspaper. Beginning on April 10, 1962, for the next fifteen months I was assigned on a permanent basis a Jeep, and was given the unfettered freedom to quite literally go where I wanted to go and come back whenever I pleased, writing about what interested me. And at the time I began my travels I was only 22 years old, having graduated Berry College less than a year earlier. It could best be described as the ultimate "dream job."

So for fifteen months every day became an adventure, every trip a vacation. I wrote well and often and anyone reading the bylines in the *Stars & Stripes* would get the impression that Sp-4 Al Provost was the only reporter at the newspaper.

There was no doubt but that possessing a Top Secret Security Clearance afforded me a leg up in this regard. Early on in this adventure I had broken down my duties into three distinctly separate areas of responsibility, as follows:

The first of these of course was that of the feature writer, whose duties are briefly discussed earlier.

The second area of responsibility was that of covering the Military Armistice Commission (MAC) meetings that were held upon demand of either the communists or the United Nations Command officials. Over the course of my 15-month tour, fourteen such meetings were held inside the Joint Security Area (JSA), and I was the only *Stars & Stripes* reporter to cover any of the meetings, that are called by either side to negotiate violations of the 1953 Armistice agreement.

During most of my 15-month tour at the *Stars & Stripes*, U.S. Air Force Maj. Gen. Joseph E. Gill was the senior member of UNC/MAC, and following each meeting I sought out General Gill for comment. His favorite (quotable) term for the communist negotiators was "predictable."

My third area of responsibility involved investigating militarily-sensitive projects that base commanders would like to appear in the *Stars & Stripes*. I was the only reporter who could possibly cover these stories because I was the only reporter who possessed a Top Secret Security Clearance.

Upon request by the base commander I would make an appointment to view the weapon. From this interview and demonstration I would write the story and take the accompanying photographs.

Upon my return to Seoul I would stop by Col. George Creel's office at U.S. Eighth Army Headquarters, located on the Yongsan compound, and hand-deliver to him my written story and all the film I had used during the demonstration. From that point it was out of my hands.

During the course of my fifteen months at the *Stars & Stripes* I investigated and reported on seven such weapons or weapons-related systems. Only one of these ever made it to the pages of the newspaper. U.S. Army censors are a heartless bunch.

My intimate knowledge of communist *North Korea* is gleaned from my second U.S. Army tour of duty that included my role as one of seven North Korean Prisoner of War interrogators stationed with Company A of the 502nd Military Intelligence Battalion (the notorious *502*) in Seoul. This tour of duty lasted for 16 months.

Sandwiched between these two eye-opening tours of duty in Korea were the 47 weeks studying the Korean language at the prestigious Defense Language Institute, located in Monterey, California, and the 8-week Prisoner of War Interrogation Course at the U.S. Army Intelligence Center, located at Ft. Holabird, in Baltimore, Maryland.

In *Memories of Distant Places* I recount my utterly fascinating experiences as a newspaper feature writer and prisoner interrogator. The story reads like an adventure movie, except that every word is true. I developed stomach ulcers during my fifth month at the infamous "502," also known as Company A, 502nd Military Intelligence Battalion. The military physicians attributed the ulcers – all seven Prisoner of War interrogators were afflicted – to the stresses associated with interrogating captured North Korean espionage agents daily for months. Two years after my honorable discharge I was still feeling the lingering effects of that malady.

In this book I discuss in detail the capture, interrogation and execution of a half-dozen North Korean espionage agents. The memoir was never intended to be a chronicle of every enemy agent I interrogated during the sixteen months I spent at the 502. This was included in order to demonstrate to the reader the realities of wartime interrogations of captured enemy spies.

Prologue

Most experiences in life are as ephemeral as a wisp of cloud on a breezy autumn afternoon. A few however, stick to you like Uncle Remus' Tar Baby, and never ever let go. Of your life. And of your soul. Take my own life, for example. And my soul. And my time spent in the notorious 502. Just writing these words "notorious 502" still elicits a laugh-cry reflex lasting several minutes. I'll try my best to control my emotions. But even after half a century, it's still hard to do. Please bear with me.

This is my second memoir. My first memoir, that recounted my life from birth on April 30, 1939 until graduation from high school in May 1957, was published in 2005 and became an overnight best seller. It was titled *Reflections in an Orphan's Eye – A Decade at Oxford 1947-1957*. A month after publication it had leapfrogged to Number 5 on the publisher's list of its Top Ten Royalty Earning Books, and remained on the coveted list for nearly a year. I was rightly proud.

Memories of Distant Places chronicles the fascinating, improbable tale of how an orphaned boy from a small town in North Carolina graduated world-renowned Berry College in 1961 with a degree in Physics-Mathematics, and a month later, at age 21 was granted a coveted Top Secret Security Clearance by the FBI. Two weeks later he enlisted in the U.S. Army, completing Basic Infantry Training and Advanced Artillery Training, then through guile and audacity, at the age of 22, wrangled a job as the sole feature writer for the *Pacific Stars and Stripes* daily newspaper in Seoul. He then parlayed this opportunity into an invitation to join U.S. Army Intelligence, where after a year of studying the Korean language and Prisoner Interrogation, he became the youngest Korean linguist and Prisoner of War interrogator at the infamous 502. Following his Honorable Discharge from the U.S. Army after four years, four months and four days, he became a licensed attorney, licensed Optometrist and the best-selling author of 16 published mystery novels and two published memoirs.

And had one helluva lot of fun along the way.

If I had my life to live all over again, I would not change it even one iota.

And that's a fact.

See amazon.com or barnesandnoble.com under A.L. PROVOST for a list of books, and visit the author at www.alprovostbooks.com.

Introduction

Korea Becomes the Two Koreas
How We Got to January 3, 1962

Korea is a nearly 600-mile-long, irregular, S-shaped peninsula, that varies in width from 125 to 200 miles. It encompasses an area about the size of Minnesota. Korea lies in the same latitudes as the eastern United States, between Maine and Georgia. In the United States, the 38th parallel runs through a line connecting Salisbury, Maryland and Fredericksburg, Virginia, roughly equidistant between Richmond, Virginia and Washington, D.C.

Korea divides the Yellow Sea to the west, from the Sea of Japan, that Koreans still call the *Tonghae*, or East Sea. Westerners refer to the country as "Korea." The name was derived from the Koryo dynasty (AD 918 to 1392), that translates as "High and Beautiful." Today many North Koreans continue to use *Choson*, the dynasty that ruled from 1392 to 1910, and many South Koreans use *Taehan*, as the official name of their country.

Korea's religious, legal and social structure have been influenced for the most part, by China. Despite its cultural ties with the Chinese people however, Korea developed its own distinct identity. The Koreans are a "pure" race. An astute Westerner, having spent a few days with a Japanese, Chinese and Korean, is able from that day forward, to distinguish among the three races.

In 1443, near the beginning of the *Choson* dynasty, the Korean phonetic alphabet, called *Hangul*, was completed under the direction of King Sejong. As a result, a Korean living in Pusan, the port city situated on the southern tip of Korea, is able to converse freely with a Korean who lives on the banks of the Yalu River, that divides Korea and China. Unlike the Soviet Union and China, there are no distinctly separate dialects, or languages, among the Korean people. Korean is Korean is Korean, as the saying goes.

In 1905 Japan invaded Korea, and for thirty-six years, from 1910 until the end of World War II, Japan ruled Korea as a Japanese colony. The root cause of present-day Korean problems, both North and South, can be traced directly to the warmongering Japanese in 1905.

The Cairo Declaration, issued on December 1, 1943 by the United States, Great Britain and China, pledged that, "in due course," Korea would have its independence.

Following the Potsdam Conference in July 1945, the victorious Allies issued the *Potsdam Declaration*, that reiterated the validity of the 1943 *Cairo Declaration*.

On August 8, 1945, the Soviet Union entered the war against Japan, at which time Joseph Stalin pledged to support the independence of Korea. The wily Stalin, however, recognized an opportunity to exert Soviet influence over the Far East.

On October 14, 1945, when Stalin's hand-picked puppet, Kim Il Sung, arrived in Pyongyang, he was wearing the uniform of a major in the Red Army. He was introduced to the people of Pyongyang as a national hero.

The infamous *38th Parallel* never was intended to be an international boundary. On August 11, 1945 the United States drafted General Order No. 1, that included the terms of Japanese surrender in Korea.

The Order provided that Japanese forces *north* of latitude 38 degrees north, the 38th Parallel, would surrender to the Soviets, and those *south* of that line, to the Americans. Stalin did not object to this Order. On September 9, 1945, the United States received the Japanese surrender in Seoul.

The designation of the 38th Parallel was made for purposes of convenience only. After all, *somebody* had to accept the surrender of thousands of Japanese troops, and do so in some order.

Thus began the story of the *Two Koreas*. On September 8, 1945, when American troops first landed in the *southern* part of Korea, Soviet forces had already been in the *northern* part of Korea for a month.

By the following day, September 9, 1945, when the United States received the Japanese surrender in Seoul, Soviet forces had already begun sealing off the 38th Parallel. Almost overnight, the world was introduced to *North* Korea and *South* Korea. Soviet occupation forces had quickly turned what had been intended only as a line of administrative convenience on a Hammond map of the world, into what, through no official action, treaty or agreement, was to become an *international boundary*. This artificial border was practically indefensible.

The Democratic People's Republic of Korea (DPRK) was proclaimed on September 9, 1948, under the dictatorship of Premier Kim Il Sung. The Republic of Korea (ROK) was proclaimed on August 15, 1948, with President Syngman Rhee as its leader. North Korea boasted heavy machinery, mineral resources, and electric power. South Korea had a larger population, light industry, and a broad agricultural base. An immediate and detrimental consequence of the division of Korea was the fact that only *twenty percent* of the land area of North Korea will support agriculture.

On June 25, 1950, the North Korean Army invaded South Korea, quickly overrunning the inept South Korean mainly defensive force of 98,000 men. On September 15, 1950, aided by record thirty-foot-high tides, General Douglas MacArthur counterattacked, outflanking the North Korean Army via amphibious landings at Inchon, on the west coast of South Korea.

General MacArthur's bold move caught the overextended North Korean Army completely by surprise. The communist invasion forces were trapped, and either surrendered, or fled northward. By October 1, 1950, only three months after the invasion, United Nations forces, led by the United States, were back at the 38th Parallel. The communists' stroll through the park was over.

On September 27, 1950, the U.S. Joint Chiefs of Staff ordered General MacArthur to destroy the North Korean armed forces, and two days later, President Truman authorized MacArthur to advance into North Korea, a move that was approved by the United Nations General Assembly on October 7, 1950. On October 20, 1950, U.N. forces entered Pyongyang, the capital of North Korea, and on October 26, 1950, American forces reached the Chinese border at the Yalu River.

Mao Zedong, known also to a generation of American schoolchildren born in the forties and fifties, as "Mao Tse-tung," who had wanted no part in Kim Il Sung's folly, also could not tolerate General Douglas MacArthur peering across the Yalu River through a pair of powerful

U.S. Army field binoculars. So the order emanated from Beijing, at the time called "Peking," and in November 1950, the Yellow Horde attacked in overwhelming force across the Yalu.

However, the Chinese army's advance came to a screeching halt near Pyongtaek, about thirty miles south of Seoul, its numbers decimated by U.S. M-60 machine guns and 155mm howitzers, giving new meaning to the military expression, "cannon fodder."

In February 1952 the U.N. General Assembly formally condemned China as an aggressor. By March 31, 1952, U.N. forces had again reached the 38th Parallel.

China's Mao Zedong resented being drawn into the war by the wiles and deceit of Kim Il Sung and Joseph Stalin. China committed troops to North Korea only after the Americans had reached the Yalu River and Mao Zedong believed China would be invaded by the riled-up General Douglas MacArthur.

Mao Zedong's fears proved to be founded in fact. In March 1952, General MacArthur publicly advocated extending the war into China, as payback for China's intervention in Korea.

However, President Truman, committing the bigger blunder of his administration, dismissed MacArthur, because of the latter's impudence, and replaced America's All-time No. 1 Hero, with the lukewarm General Matthew B. Ridgeway. "Matt" did the best he could, operating without a clear mandate to win the war.

The Korean War ended in a costly stalemate, with the Armistice that was signed on July 27, 1953. Kim Il Sung and Joseph Stalin's stupid gamble had resulted in roughly four million casualties, the brunt of which were suffered by North Korea and China. North Korea never would have started the Korean War without the backing of the Soviet Union. The Chinese certainly had not encouraged Kim Il Sung; Mao Zedong sought no argument with the Americans.

China had been the biggest loser, having been "suckered" into a war that it had not started, and in which it wanted no part. South Korean casualties were 1,313,000 including 1,000,000 civilians. North Korean casualties were estimated at 2,500,000 including 1,000,000 civilians. Military *deaths* included, United States (33,629), South Korea (47,000), U.N. forces (3,194), and North Korea (520,000).

The foregoing discussion provides an overview of Korea through the date of the signing of the Armistice, July 27, 1953.

After the Armistice – Turmoil

Following the signing of the Armistice, South Korea enjoyed a postwar boom in education, and school enrollment increased at a rapid pace. By 1960 more than seventy percent of the population could read and write. That year, Tong-a Ilbo, South Korea's largest newspaper, boasted a circulation in excess of 400,000 readers.

However as President Syngman Rhee was to discover, an educated population is a much less tolerant population.

Syngman Rhee had been president of the Republic of Korea (ROK) since 1949. In reality Rhee was little more than a petty dictator, who single-handedly controlled the nation through a corrupt military and bureaucracy. The economy struggled.

Into this quagmire of abuse of power stepped thousands of college students. During the late fifties opposition groups formed, and by 1960, bloodied but determined, well-organized student protests filled the streets of Seoul.

In May 1960, a year before I graduated from Berry College, Syngman Rhee, realizing his days in power likely were numbered in the single digits, resigned the presidency and departed for Hawaii, leaving an impotent government floating in the Sea of Japan without a rudder.

In July 1960 the South Korean constitution was changed to form a new government, one in which the cabinet would be responsible to the legislature.

Yun Po Son was elected President of the *Second Republic*, and Chang Mi You was installed as Prime Minister.

However Yun and Chang could not get along, and the political situation worsened. The final break came nearly a year later when in May 1961, the month I graduated from Berry College, Prime Minister Chang announced his intention to *cut 30,000 military positions*. Throughout the world, the military does not tend to react favorably when faced with such threats.

My Role in the History of the Two Koreas
May 15, 1961-November 4, 1965

On *May 15, 1961*, I graduated Berry College with a degree in Physics-Mathematics. The following day, *May 16, 1961*, Kim Jong Pil, a young lieutenant colonel in the South Korean Army, and his uncle-by-marriage, General Park Chung Hee, took control of a floundering South Korean government in a lightning but bloodless coup. The previous year the three-term president, the corrupt Syngman Rhee had resigned the presidency and quickly fled to Honolulu, Hawaii, leaving behind an inept government, believed by North Korea to be "ripe for the taking."

General Park moved quickly to solidify his control of the country. In June 1961, a month after he took control, fearing a military threat from North Korea, General Park dissolved the South Korean National Assembly.

Simultaneously the general formed a military junta, called the Supreme Council for National Reconstruction (SCNR). Martial law was declared, and a midnight-dawn curfew was put into effect. Vehicles on the road after dark were required to have lights on *inside* the vehicles. Martial law was lifted in 1962, however the midnight-dawn curfew remained in effect.

On *June 1, 1961* I applied to the FBI, seeking a position as a Special Agent. The Special Agent who interviewed me at FBI headquarters in Washington, D.C. informed me that the FBI would perform a background check, then call me in for a second interview within two weeks.

This second interview took place on *June 14, 1961*. I declined the offer of employment because as a person could not become a Special Agent until reaching age 25, I would have to work in the FBI Crime Lab for longer than two years, until age 25. To me, this was a waste of two years.

However unbeknown to me at the time, the FBI had investigated my background and had awarded me a coveted *Top Secret Security Clearance.*

On *June 30, 1961* I enlisted in the U.S. Army, with a goal in mind of attending Officer Candidate School (OCS) in Artillery, at Ft. Sill, Oklahoma, after completing Basic Infantry Training at Ft. Jackson, South Carolina in the fall of 1961.

This turn of events set up what was to become a confusing situation that would follow me throughout my U.S. Army career.

The salient facts are as follows: Security Clearances are awarded by the FBI, not by the U.S. Army. The highest security clearance awarded was the *Top Secret Security Clearance*. Even members of the U.S. Congress are not awarded Top Secret Clearances absent good cause. Nor are generals in the U.S. Army automatically given Top Secret Clearances. At the time, I was likely one of the few 22-year-olds in the United States who possessed a Top Secret Security Clearance.

What really stumped high-ranking, envious army officers was the following:

At the time I was awarded a Top Secret Security Clearance, *June 14, 1961*, I was not employed by the FBI, and had not enlisted in the U.S. Army. This apparent anomaly was to crop up more than two dozen times during my army career, that spanned 4 years, 4 months and 4 days. The problem was exacerbated by my absolute refusal to explain or discuss the unique situation.

On September 2, 1961 I completed the 8-week Basic Infantry Training Course at Ft. Jackson, South Carolina, then went directly to Ft. Sill, Oklahoma to begin the 8-week Advanced Artillery Training Course.

Following completion of training on the 105mm Howitzer I found myself in limbo until the next Artillery Officer Candidate School began classes in December 1961.

This is the point at which I was informed that in order to be accepted into OCS I would have had to re-enlist in the army for another three years. I balked at this requirement, opted out of OCS and a week later began a 28-day ocean voyage to Korea.

Adultery on the High Seas

My mother's love for my sister Eoline, two years older than I, my brother Pete, four years my junior, and I, only deepened as we three children grew up at Oxford Orphanage. Mom attended our high school graduation, Eoline's graduation from Nursing School and my graduation from Berry College in May 1961.

In 1958 at the age of 61, my mother suffered her first of two strokes, that was followed by a gradual decline in her health.

There were perhaps a dozen or more *dependents*, wives and children of military officers, who had hitched a ride on the thousand-man troopship as far as Honolulu, where they would rejoin husbands stationed in Hawaii.

These dependents were separated from the U.S. Army troops by a simple hemp cord, but the two groups, troops and dependents, could talk to one another freely. Which is apparently what happened. The deck of the ship was patrolled by U.S. Navy personnel, and the dependents were confined to an area of the deck forward of midships.

The entire deck of the ship was cleared of all personnel at 9:00 p.m. On the fourth night out the U.S. Navy patrol discovered a female dependent, a wife, and a U.S. soldier on his way to Korea, engaged in sex behind one of the huge exhaust fans on the dependents' side of the rope barrier, while the woman's three small children were inside their cabin below deck.

The woman and her children were confined to quarters for the three days it took to reach Honolulu. The adulterous G.I. was confined to the brig during this period.

The scheduled call at the port of Honolulu was to take on fuel, food and supplies. However all hands – the thousand G.I.s, the ship's crew and the dependents – were called on deck to witness the shame suffered by the cuckolded U.S. Army captain waiting on shore.

First the woman and her three children were escorted off the ship to her husband.

Next more than a thousand men watched as the handcuffed soldier-adulterer-prisoner was led off the ship by a U.S. Navy Shore Patrol.

This drama unfolded during the month of December 1961. The adulterous G.I. would be given a dishonorable discharge. However this would occur only after he had spent many months, and possibly years, confined to the prison at Leavenworth, Kansas.

The Army of 1961 was not the Army of 2018.

My Mother's Death

Our next port of call was Tokyo Bay. At around 3:00 p.m. on the third day before we reached Japan, the ship's captain summoned me to his quarters.

In a quite manner he informed me that my mother had passed away in a Kinston hospital the previous night. He informed me that he could summon a helicopter to pick me up and take me to the airport in Tokyo, from where I could fly to North Carolina, where my sister and five brothers would be waiting. "You give the word and I'll make the call, son," he said.

I asked the captain if I could have a few minutes to think over the situation. He said for me to take my time, picked up his service cap and exited the room.

My mother had suffered from the date of my father's death in 1946 until her own death in 1961. However she was gone, and there was nothing I could do for her. The funeral was already being held up for my sister and five brothers, and I did not wish to impose upon them.

When the captain returned I conveyed my reasoning to him. He said he respected my decision. He shook hands with me and wished me well. Sadly I returned to my group.

At the time I and 999 other deathly seasick G.I.s landed at the Port of Inchon on January 3, 1962, I had been graduated from Berry College for only seven and a half months, and my favorite dictator, General Park Chung Hee, had been in power an equal amount of time, mainly because I had graduated Berry College on May 15, 1961 and the general had assumed power in Seoul the following day, May 16, 1961. Our second, more memorable meeting, had yet to take place.

In June 1961, the same month I enlisted in the U.S. Army and began Basic Infantry Training at Ft. Jackson, South Carolina, the newly-formed SCNR established the Korean Central Intelligence Agency (KCIA). The KCIA was similar to the Soviet Union KGB, because of its blanket power base, exerting its influence in *domestic* as well as foreign affairs.

At this point allow me to digress momentarily, in order to bring the story up to date.

Chapter 1

◇◇◇◇

The Improbable Adventure Begins

I was born and spent the first seventeen years of my life in God's Country, as North Carolina is known throughout the world. Or at least in North Carolina.

Following my May 1957 graduation from high school in Kinston, a small town situated astride U.S. 70 southeast of Raleigh, I attended East Carolina College (now East Carolina University) for the 1957 Summer Term.

Eager to see just a smidgen of what the rest of the South was like, following the Summer Term I packed all my personal belongings into my 1951 black 2-door Chevrolet Power Glide and headed generally in a southerly direction, to "find my way," or "make my mark," or whatever young people do when they decide to sever all ties to an unhappy childhood and strike out on their own.

Two weeks after leaving my dear widowed mother in tears – Mom had always been quickly brought to tears – I ended my travels in the Administration Building at Berry College, a four-year college situated seven miles north of the Rome, Georgia northern city limit sign, 70 miles northwest of Atlanta.

Of the several thousand students enrolled in Berry College in the fall of 1957, I didn't know even one. Ninety percent of the students were from Georgia. Only one percent were from North Carolina.

At Berry College we ate "family-style," as opposed to "cafeteria-style," and there were no assigned seats. At supper on the very first day of classes I took one of the eight seats, and observed quickly that all the other boys at the large table appeared to be older than I. *Upperclassmen* I believe they're called.

Not understanding the reason for this arrangement, I eased out of my chair, intent on locating a seat at another table. However before I could slink away, one of the bigger (in size) of the boys spoke up.

"No, keep your seat, Freshman Boy," he said smiling. "There's no assigned seating here."

So I sat down, resolving that I would from that night forward be more careful where I chose to eat my meals. Allow me to digress for a moment. Best not to omit anything important; I'd have to add it in later and this would alter my logical continuity writing style.

On May 15, 1957 I graduated from Wheat Swamp High School near Kinston. However I only attended Wheat Swamp High for three months, from February 15 to May 15, 1957.

For three and a half years I had attended high school in the small town of Oxford, North Carolina, mainly because this is where nationally renowned Oxford Orphanage – founded in 1872 – is located. And to this day still is in operation.

But you ask, what did this Oxford Orphanage have to do with Berry College or better still with *Memories of Distant Places*?

The detailed answer to this pivotal question can be found by reading my first of seventeen published books, a 620-page, best-selling memoir entitled *Reflections in an Orphan's Eye* and subtitled *A Decade at Oxford 1947-1957*.

Two months following the publication of the memoir in 2005 the book had jumped to No. 5 on the list of the publisher's Top 10 Best Selling Books and remained near the top of the list for nearly a year. I was honored.

My father Benjamin Daniel Provost was a refrigeration engineer. During the war (1941-1945) he worked as a U.S. civil service engineer at the Cherry Point Marine Air Station, located on the coast of North Carolina.

When the war with Japan ended in August 1945, my father continued his employment at Cherry Point. Six months later, on February 6, 1946 my father died, leaving a grieving widow and seven children. Six months later all of a sudden my only sister Eoline, age nine, was taken away – to where I had no idea – and a year after my father's death, on February 15, 1947 I was taken to Oxford Orphanage where I was reunited with my sister.

At this point the only thing I care to add about my decade at Oxford Orphanage was that on the day I left, February 15, 1957, I vowed to destroy the first stupid bully to cross my path. No more of that nonsense for me.

So after being ordered by the loudmouth upperclassman to "keep my seat," I remained seated, figuring I would allow the kid to get himself into trouble. Which was exactly what the fool did.

As we ate family-style, waitresses brought a plate of food for each boy. However student workers know nothing about food portions, and when I stared down at my plate the portion of mashed potatoes was likely more than enough for two students.

Problem was, the loudmouth sitting directly across the table from me saw the (large) mound of mashed potatoes the instant I noticed it.

"That's a lot of mashed potatoes, Freshman Boy," he said matter-of-factly, his voice rising with each word spoken, to where I was firmly convinced his tone was one of derision. He was mocking me. Up to this point the older – and bigger – upperclassman had made three statements, none of which was followed by a question mark, and his increasingly loud voice had attracted the attention of several hundred students seated in the large dining hall, who apparently had sensed trouble abrewing and had suddenly become very quiet.

Not having received an answer to a question he had not asked, the boy apparently felt some need to fill the void of silence. "Well, Freshman Boy, why don't I just sit here and make sure you eat all them mashed potatoes," he said. "What's your name anyway?"

At this point I stood up, a move that placed me looking down at him. This was an action he apparently had not counted on. He reflexively stood and we faced one another across the table like a couple of Wild West gunslingers.

"My name's Al Provost," I said evenly. "I didn't ask for all those mashed potatoes, so I'm not going to eat *any* of them. I'll give you ten seconds to start making me eat all those mashed potatoes, or else I'm leaving here. It's up to you."

You could have heard a pin drop in that crowded dining hall that night in early September 1957. For about ten seconds the bully and I stared into each other's face. Neither of us spoke. Neither of us moved.

"I didn't think so," I said evenly, not raising my voice. Then I calmly turned and slowly walked out of the dining hall.

A month later I was unanimously elected President of the Freshman Class. And I had not even sought the office.

The Mountain Day Quarterback

At Berry College there were two large literary societies, the Georgians and the Syrrebs ("Berrys" spelled backwards). Homecoming was in mid-October. The highlight of homecoming was a touch football game between the Georgians and Syrrebs. It was an annual "grudge match."

A week after humiliating the stupid dining hall loudmouth, I was approached by Don Norman, a senior and the president of the Georgians.

"We all saw what you did in the dining hall," he said, smiling and extending his hand it seemed to me, in congratulations and respect. We shook hands.

"We Georgians are in a somewhat of a bind," he began. "The homecoming football game is in six weeks, and our quarterback graduated last year."

"I played quarterback for four years in high school," I told him (truthfully) before he could continue.

"Would I be the only quarterback, or just the backup?" I asked.

"You'd be the only one. You'll find that very few of these boys have ever played high school football. So you'll just have to find three or four pass receivers and do the best you can."

Thanks a lot Don Norman, I said (under my breath).

Well I did the best I could, and in doing so also became the *coach* of the Georgians. We practiced every afternoon and I thought our chances were good.

There was only one small problem. On Mountain Day, that was what we called Homecoming, several hundred students were crowded around the football field.

First the game began. The Georgians struck first with a long pass from me to Randall Kent at the beginning of the second quarter.

Then, at about the end of the first half, with the Georgians ahead 6-0, the rain began. And there went the ball game.

I could get the ball to my receivers but none of them could hold on to the slippery pigskin. But we Georgians held the Syrrebs scoreless and at halftime we led 6-0.

And there the score remained until right at the end of the game the Syrrebs scored twice and the final score was Syrrebs 14, Georgians 6.

Thus up to that point in my brief college career I had "called out" a campus bully, quarterbacked the Georgians to a not too embarrassing close loss in the Mountain Day game, and had been elected President of the Freshman Class. The write-up in the yearbook, *The Cabin Log*, noted my touchdown pass and outstanding play, that only served to enhance my image among the students.

From the yearbook *The Log*:

> The annual Mountain Day football game saw the Syrreb Literary Society win over the Georgia Literary Society by a score of 14-6.
>
> The Georgians led at halftime 6-0 by virtue of an Al Provost to Randall Kent touchdown pass in the second period. Targets for Provost's passes during the game were Danny Coleman, David Wilson, Jerry Ward and Tommy Gammon.
>
> This passing attack proved not to be enough as the Syrrebs roared back in the second half to push the Georgians into defeat. Jim Pettigrew, Lowell Loadholtz and William Burkhalter were outstanding in the Georgia line play.

The Physics Majors

Dr. Lawrence W. McAllister was a member of the scientific team that developed the charcoal gas mask during World War I.

The brilliant physicist was also head of the Physics Department at Berry College for many decades, including my four years at Berry.

We began our Freshman year with at least fifty aspiring physics majors, and immediately encountered a giant speed bump. Even today I recall the first day of class. All physics is, said "Dr. Mac," is applied mathematics, so if you are getting a *major* in physics you must also get *major* and not a minor, in mathematics. Damn!

Anyway we lost at least a quarter of the physics hopefuls before we had barely gotten started, and many others along the way until at graduation in May 1961 only nine physics majors graduated. It was tough, but we were a close-knit group and supported one another. Following graduation we went our separate ways.

One of our group was Ann Fite. After graduation Ann married John Whitaker, another of the "band of nine." Ann and I were close friends and she was exceptionally intelligent.

In the 1961 college yearbook, the *Cabin Log* on page 23 is a photograph showing three students seated at the snack counter inside the campus bookstore.

I am the closest to the camera. The farthest away is Aaron Ellis, and seated beside me is Ann Fite. The caption above the photograph reads:

Physics majors…the bar's best customers

As I noted above we physics majors were a close-knit group and the bookstore snack bar was our favorite watering hole.

We graduated Berry College in May 1961. Sixteen years later an article in the *Miami Herald* caught my attention. The article was titled:

Two Space Flight Finalists Selected;
Woman Bypassed

The article reads in part:

> Washington – Two Pennsylvania-born scientists are finalists for seats in a U.S.-European space flight planned in 1980.
>
> They were selected by the space agency yesterday from among six candidates named last year. Among those dropped was an Alabama physicist Mrs. Ann Fite Whitaker, 38, who might have become the first American woman in space.

At the time of the 1977 newspaper article there was a good deal of speculation surrounding Ann not making the astronaut cut. One thought among our classmates was that at the time the article appeared in the newspaper in 1977, Ann was 38 years old. Because the projected date of the space flight was 1980, Ann would have been 41 or 42 years old, and the Americans had very little if any experience with a 42-year-old female in space. How unfortunate.

We nine physics majors were smart, just a wee bit on the vain side, and any one of us could have become an astronaut if he or she had elected to follow that path.

The Ultimate College Honor

Following my being voted President of the Freshman Class, although I had never sought the office, I remained until graduation a member of the student government at Berry College.

I served as Freshman Representative to the Men's Student Government, Treasurer of the Sophomore Class, Secretary, Vice-President and finally President of the Men's Student Government, in my senior year.

Miss May Parish was a Professor of Social Science at Berry. In 1960, during my Junior year Miss Parish established the Jessie Pritchett Parish Student Government Award, open to any member of the student body regardless of class. The award was established in honor of Miss Parish's mother.

At the end of my Junior year in May 1960, an assembly of the entire student body was held inside the chapel on the Ford Campus, where the female students resided.

During the awards ceremony Miss Parish read the presentation of the award. Then she announced the recipient of the first ever Jessie Pritchett Parish Student Government Award. I could hardly believe it when Miss Parish asked me to stand. The applause began without any word from Miss Parish. I was deeply honored by the Award. Not bad for a kid who had spent a decade in an orphanage.

The Award reads, in part:

> The Award goes to the person adjudged to have made, during the current school year, the greatest contribution in civil responsibility toward the cause of student government and constructive college activities in general.
>
> It is to me a real pleasure to announce at this time in behalf of the donor, the recipient of this award for the current year.
>
> Al Provost, will you please stand.

The office of President of the Men's Student Government and recipient of the Jessie Pritchett Parish Student Government Award were the ultimate honors awarded to any student at Berry College. I had received both.

In the fall of 1957 I was accepted as a Freshman at Berry College. I intended to work hard, study hard and make good grades. I had absolutely no desire to "make waves" of any kind or to become involved in campus politics. Far from it.

But I had lived at Oxford Orphanage for a full decade (February 1947 – February 1957), and had absolutely no intention of allowing any loudmouth upperclassman to insult, harass or intimidate me in front of several hundred students. Calling him out on my first day at Berry had thrust me into the spotlight and I had become the BMOC (Big Man on Campus).

I firmly believe that my life has been defined by a number of seminal moments. As an example, imagine how my life would have turned out if the student food server had served me a smaller portion of mashed potatoes that fateful first night at Berry College?

During my encounter with the stupid upperclassman in the dining hall, he had asked me my name. I told him my name was Al Provost, then in the same breath challenged him "to put up or shut up." So several hundred students had learned on my very first day at Berry that I was not one to back down from a bully. This engendered almost instant trust and respect among the students.

I passed through four years as a student at Berry College clothed in a coat of modesty. Of the offices I held on campus I had never campaigned for any of them. I never had a "best friend" among the students but I'm certain that in my senior year I knew every student at Berry College on a first-name basis.

Origin of the Top Secret Security Clearance

In my senior year I applied to the Physics Department at the University of Georgia in Athens. I intended to work toward a Masters Degree and then a Doctorate in Atomic Physics.

In February 1961, three months prior to graduation, I received a Letter of Acceptance from the Dean of the Physics Department at UGA. The university offered a stipend of $1600 per calendar year, with the stipulation that I teach a freshman physics course during both the fall and spring semesters.

A few drawbacks came with this offer of acceptance. When I graduated from Berry College in May 1961 I did not own an automobile. If we divide $1600 by twelve months we get $134 per month. The only way I could survive financially would be if I worked a full-time night job.

I have been as successful in life as I have by abiding by one strict unwavering rule: *Know thyself.* From my decade growing up at Oxford Orphanage I learned to live within my financial means. Don't borrow money that I can't pay back. *Knowing oneself* means knowing your limitations and living within them.

Having made my decision to forego the teaching assistantship, I wrote a nice letter to the university, thanking the head of the Physics Department for his consideration, while declining the offer.

Two weeks following the May 1961 graduation I borrowed my older brother Doc's automobile – he lived in Bethesda, Maryland, just outside Washington, D.C. – and drove down to FBI headquarters. I explained to the receptionist that I had come to inquire about the position of Special Agent. Ten minutes later I was seated at a large table in the conference room across from a Special Agent.

I had brought with me a transcript of my Berry College grades, the Letter of Acceptance from the Physics Department Dean at UGA, my 1961 Berry College yearbook and a copy of my Jessie Pritchett Parish Student Government Award.

The FBI Special Agent interviewed me for about thirty minutes, then made a copy of my fingerprints. He said the FBI would perform a background check and that he would telephone me within two weeks to set up a second interview.

We all know what Yogi Berra said about déjà vu. This occurred on my second interview with the special agent. He explained that the FBI wanted to offer me the position of Special Agent. However this could not occur under the existing FBI rules, that provided that an applicant must be at least 25 years old before he or she could become a Special Agent. And I had just reached age 22. So what would I do for the next three years? Anticipating my question, the Special Agent explained.

I would join the FBI and work in the FBI Crime Laboratory for two and a half years, until age twenty-four and a half. Then the FBI would waive the last six months of the age requirement and I would become a Special Agent at age twenty-four and a half.

Sounds like a winner, I thought. By the way I said, what will be my salary for the next two and a half years?

You'll come in as a Crime Lab Technician, said the Special Agent. That's a GS-4.

And what is the salary of a GS-4, I asked.

It's $4,000 per year, he said.

And the déjà vu bug had struck again. Quickly dividing $4,000 by twelve months, I came up with $333 per month.

Again I was just out of college and still didn't own an automobile. The lab technician position was a full-time, 8-to-5 job. So I would have to get a part-time or full-time night job just to make ends meet for the next two and a half years. All things considered, I couldn't do it.

I relate this story for the following reason, one that at the time was not all that important. In order for the FBI to have offered me a job they must have performed a thorough background check on me, that resulted in some degree of Security Clearance, namely *Confidential*, *Secret* or *Top Secret*, which is the highest Security Clearance. This fact will become clear later on in my story.

Several days after my second meeting with the Special Agent I telephoned FBI headquarters. I reluctantly declined the offer, and he wished me well in my future endeavors.

However apparently the FBI believed I would accept the offer of employment. Therefore the FBI awarded me a *Top Secret Security Clearance*, an act that would prove confusing to some persons on down the road. The timeline went something like this:

On May 15, 1961 I graduated from Berry College. I had turned 22 just two weeks earlier.

On June 1, 1961 I applied to the FBI for a position as a Special Agent, and underwent an interview.

On June 14, 1961 the FBI offered me employment as a Crime Lab Technician. I declined the offer.

I joined the U.S. Army on June 30, 1961.

Therefore as of the date of being awarded the Top Secret Security Clearance, that is, about June 10, 1961, I did not work for the FBI and was not in the U.S. Army.

Furthermore once the FBI had granted me the Top Secret Security Clearance, there was no reason to rescind the award.

I included the foregoing passage because it explains the reason for my *Top Secret Security Clearance* and its significance to the overall story.

Even though I declined the FBI's offer of employment, still the FBI had performed a background check, and believing I would accept their offer of employment, awarded me a *Top Secret Security Clearance*, although I was not aware of this fact at the time.

Chapter 2

◇◇◇◇

I Enlist in the U.S. Army – The Adventure Begins

In mid-June 1961 I spoke with the U.S. Army recruiter in Baltimore. He assured me that I would be able to attend Officer Candidate School (OCS) in Artillery after undergoing Basic Infantry Training at Ft. Jackson, South Carolina and Advanced Artillery Training at Ft. Sill, Oklahoma.

However the Army recruiter neglected to mention the famous *Caveat*.

So after completing Basic Infantry Training and Advanced Artillery Training I was told to just hang around the company, in limbo so to speak, until the next Artillery OCS class formed.

A week or so later Captain John Corning, the company commander, called me into his office. He explained to me what the Army recruiter had neglected to tell me before I enlisted.

I did not intend making the army a career. The regular enlistment was for three years. However the rule was that there had to be at least three years *remaining* on my enlistment *after* completing OCS. In other words I would be required to re-enlist for an additional three years if I desired to attend Officer Candidate School.

Captain Corning placed a sheet of paper on the desk in front of me. There were boxes to be checked. One box indicated that the candidate agreed to re-enlist for an additional three years. The second box indicated that I declined entry into OCS. I checked the second box and signed my name.

A month later I boarded a troopship in Oakland, California along with a thousand other G.I.s bound for Korea via Honolulu and Tokyo. The voyage took twenty-eight days. I was violently seasick for twenty-eight days. So were the other thousand unlucky G.I.s on that damned death ship.

On January 3, 1962 we arrived at the processing center at the port of Inchon, forty miles west of Seoul, the capital of South Korea. The following morning some fifty of us boarded a Korean passenger train for the day-long trip to Chunchon, the home of Camp Page and the U.S. Army's Fourth Missile Command.

The mission of the Fourth Missile Command was to defend northern South Korea during war by deploying the surface-to-surface Honest John Rocket, considered state-of-the art but even at that time was not all that accurate or reliable. Trust me, I know of what I speak. It was fin-stabilized and the scatter-on-target was out of sight, for starters.

One place you never want to be in January and February is Korea. Bitterly cold days on end, made even worse because the months of January, February and March are part of the rainy season in Korea.

When the sergeant read off the names of the *Unfortunate 50* destined for the slow train ride inside a Korean passenger train devoid of heat, we had to grab our duffel bags and slog through ankle-deep mud just to reach the deuce-and-a-half (a two and a half ton truck) for the ride across Inchon to the train depot.

The soldiers riding in the huge troop carrier kept looking at one another, not saying a word. Not even the hint of a smile among the half-hundred men. Nobody spoke. Silently we were all asking the same unanswerable question: What in the hell have I gotten myself into?

Moreover more bad news awaited us upon the Korean train's arrival at the Chunchon train depot. The train dropped us off and continued on its route. We stood in a freezing rain for two hours until another deuce and a half lumbered along.

While undergoing Advanced Artillery Training at Ft. Sill, Oklahoma in the winter of 1961 I had trained on the 105mm Howitzer, an extremely accurate – in the right hands that is – cannon that fires shells at a high trajectory.

However whether the cannon is a large Honest John Rocket or a small (by comparison) 105mm Howitzer, the theory of the projectile's flight is nearly the same. Thus because my test scores on the 105mm Howitzer were high, I suppose the Army figured I could quickly master the operation of the awesome Honest John, my degree in Physics-Mathematics likely having some bearing on the Army's decision to send me to that frozen tundra called Korea.

The large truck rolled across Chunchon and entered through the front gate of Camp Page. It turned left on the first narrow street and stopped in front of a series of Quonset huts, that pass for military barracks in some parts of the world.

A Quonset hut is a prefabricated metal shelter like a half cylinder lying on its flat side. The vast majority of buildings constructed on U.S. military posts in Korea were gray Quonset huts, including those in Panmunjom where the Military Armistice Commission meetings were held.

The only thing wrong with that picture was that nobody was there to meet the new arrivals. So the *Unfortunate 50* piled off the truck and stood milling about in small groups waiting for some sort of guidance.

Finally a Master Sergeant came out of one of the Quonset huts. He told us to "fall in," then gave us the bad news.

The previous day our company had begun a fifteen-day training exercise. We were to eat supper in the mess hall, then be shown to our Quonset huts. After breakfast the following morning someone would drive us to the site of the maneuvers.

"How long will these maneuvers last?" queried one of the newcomers rather hesitantly. "Two weeks," came the sergeant's reply.

"Will we return to base at night?" (Hesitantly.)

"No." (Firmly.)

"You mean we'll have to sleep in tents at night?" (Indignantly.)

"Yes. But because we'll be under combat conditions we'll move to a new location every other night."

"How long does a move take?"

"Most of the night."

"But Sarge, we've been on a goddam troopship for twenty-eight days and we're sick as dogs. When are we going to get some rest?"

The sergeant empathized with our plight. However he did not make the rules. Finally, his patience seeming to wear just a wee bit thin, the young Private sensed this and decided it might be more prudent not to ask any more stupid questions.

Following a welcomed supper, a restless sleep and a morning breakfast, we loaded up two trucks with all our gear and headed out in search of our company. Reluctantly of course. And in the freezing rain of course.

Critical Decisions

On the four-hour drive to our unit in the mountains of northeast Korea I made several decisions. First of all it disturbed me to no end to think that I might spend the next year at Camp Page in the mountains. An entire year in that godforsaken place? No way in hell would I do this. All I had to do was think my way out of this dilemma. I had spent ten years of my childhood outfoxing the adult staff of 346-child Oxford Orphanage in North Carolina following my father's death. This would be no different. The opportunity would present itself. I just had to be prepared, to start making my own luck. Oxford Orphanage had been a training ground for the perils of life.

The second thing I refused to do was to live for a year in a country of thirteen million Orientals and not be able to speak their language. I was smarter than the average man. Learning the Korean language couldn't really be all that difficult, could it? Well, could it? When these two weeks of misery were over I would ask someone at headquarters for guidance. But first things first. And the most pressing problem at the moment was how to keep out of this freezing rain for the next two weeks.

My company was charged with setting up and operating the Field Headquarters for the Fourth U.S. Missile Command, a large camouflaged brown van. To further avoid detection by the communist North Koreans, this van was positioned in one of the lowest elevations in the area.

The entire two-week exercise under real conditions was controlled from this large van. The actual physical location of the Honest John Rockets was many miles away, in Camp Kaiser.

I didn't mind dodging freezing raindrops during the day. But I had to find a way to keep out of the elements at night.

In 1962 enlisted men (EM) in the U.S. Army were rarely college graduates. Especially one with an undergraduate degree in Physics. With a specialty in *Rocketry*, as I divulged to a major early on the first morning at the Field Headquarters site. Was there any way I could help?

Of course I was stretching the "Rocketry" angle a bit, but I figured it fitted in with the degree in Physics, that was easily proved just by glancing at my personnel folder or "jacket" as it was called.

Simulated firings of the huge Honest John Rocket certainly would not be carried out at night, so the only thing needed in the Headquarters van was an intelligent enlisted man to answer the telephone – if it ever rang – and pass on any messages or orders to the officers asleep in the nearby large heated tents.

So for twelve days I manned the perimeter with my trust 9.5-pound M1 Garand rifle, crouched in foxholes that had been dug years before, and defended the Headquarters van from attack by an imaginary communist infantry assault. In twelve days the Commies never once succeeded in breaching our perimeter. We were good!

As noted above the five officers controlling the Rocket deployment called it a night at 10:00 p.m. The major gave me my orders re answering the field telephones and I was left alone in the huge van.

Before the mess hall kitchen closed for the night the company cook brought over a pot of fresh coffee, a burner and plenty of sandwiches. I thanked him profusely.

Very few calls came in during those twelve nights and truth be told the calls I did answer likely were to see whether all of us had gone to sleep. Very comfortable, safe and thoroughly uneventful nights.

I had been alone in the huge van for an hour or so when suddenly I became bored. So I opened a footlocker resting on a fold-up card table in the corner and withdrew several U.S. Army Technical Manuals that covered the operation of the Honest John Rocket. Some officer had neglected to padlock the footlocker.

Back when I had applied to attend OCS the FBI had investigated my background and I possessed a *Top Secret Security Clearance.* So I withdrew one of the technical manuals, poured myself a large mug of hot coffee and began reading.

I had studied mechanics as part of my Physics curriculum at Berry College, so I possessed a fairly detailed understanding of Rocketry. This knowledge was enhanced by studying the Theory of Trajectory as part of my 8-week Advanced Artillery Training at Ft. Sill, Oklahoma prior to being forced at the tip of a bayonet to board that damned deathtrap of a troopship in Oakland, California.

Daring Escape from Camp Page

After twelve days we returned to Camp Page, thankful that we didn't have to lug those heavy 9.5-pound M1 rifles around with us all day long. The first thing I did after breakfast was to visit the Headquarters Day Room to study the messages on the corkboard attached to the wall. I was searching for *anything* that would help get me the hell out of the following year's misery called Camp Page, as well as information on learning the Korean language. And again I was making my own luck, not depending on some Guardian Angel to do it for me. Perseverance would pay off.

My study of the Korean language was delayed somewhat by the fact that for the next two months we spent on ten-day or twelve-day training maneuvers.

And things weren't going all that smoothly with the cantankerous Honest John simulated firings. One Saturday morning we all had to fall out in formation while our camp commandant, a colonel, was supposed to conduct a test firing for the benefit of several South Korean Army generals. After two frustrating hours the colonel called it quits. C'est la vie at Camp Page, Korea in 1962.

American soldiers seem to be constantly bombarded by training films. I should know. In my four and a half years in the Army I served on *seven* different Army posts. We were always watching films. And films are shown by the use of projectors. And these several types of projectors need real live operators to show the films. These operators are called "projectionists." And lo and behold guess who needed a full-time projectionist? You're correct. *Camp Page*. The note on the 5x8 card thumbtacked to the Message Board indicated that anyone interested should just walk down to the film building and ask around.

Suddenly I had stumbled upon my ticket out of the hellhole called Chunchon. And instantly I took measures to secure my decision to become Camp Page's *only* projectionist – I reached up, snatched the 5x8 card off the bulletin board, folded it twice, stuffed it into my pocket and walked away. Later, when no one else was around I would tear the stupid 5x8 card into 28,317 pieces, small.

Finding someone to teach me Korean would have to wait an hour or two. I stopped by the large snack shop on base, that was operated by Koreans, ordered two large chocolate milk shakes and headed down to the large film building situated at the edge of the base.

In my desperation to escape Camp Page I certainly was not above offering a bribe, and it turned out that the thirsty projectionist was not above accepting one. So we sat and slurped our shakes while he explained why he needed a projectionist and how I would go about it if I just happened to be interested.

Fifteen minutes later we agreed that in the event I could not escape from Camp Page the next best thing would be to become the base projectionist. He would be leaving for his return stateside in ten days, which would give me time to take the Korean train to Seoul to attend the week-long projectionist course.

Seems as though being the base projectionist was a full-time job. He showed the films inside a large theatre on base and was his own boss. He kept the only key to the film building. My kind of job.

Early the next morning I boarded the Korean train for the four-hour trip to Seoul.

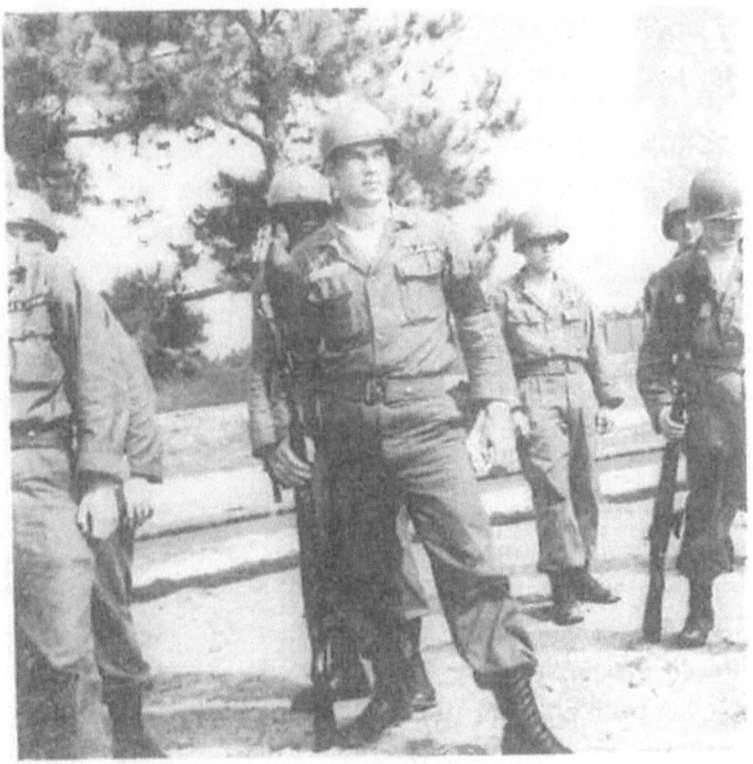

July and August 1961. Basic Infantry Training, Ft. Jackson, South Carolina. Waiting my turn on the firing line with my trusty 9.5-pound Ml Garand firle. The black armband on my left arm identifies me as one of my platoon's four squad leaders I was later awarded a Marksman's Badge.

Chapter 3

◇◇◇◇

A Most Fortuitous Conversation

I arrived at the Seoul Train Depot in mid-afternoon Saturday, and took a Korean taxi to Eighth U.S. Army Headquarters located in the Yongsan District of Seoul. I showed a copy of my orders to attend Projectionist School to the Duty Sergeant. He issued me bedding in the Transient Quarters and told me where the Mess Hall was located.

I've never been a smoker and any form of alcohol gives me instant heartburn. But just to kill a few hours I located the first bar within walking distance of the Yongsan Compound. I entered, sat at the bar and ordered a Coke.

And overheard a most interesting conversation. Unforgettable, it was.

As I recall that late afternoon, the bar was somewhat crowded. There was an unoccupied barstool directly on my left. However on the barstool directly to my right sat an American. He was dressed in civilian clothes, and was carrying on a conversation with a sergeant seated to his immediate right who was dressed in his uniform.

Now in 1962 American soldiers off base still had to wear their uniform. So who was the man seated to my right? Soldier? Or civilian?

I could even today quite likely render a verbatim account of the conversation. In the interest of clarity however, allow me to simply give you the gist of what transpired. Absolutely fascinating encounter.

There must have been at least a half-dozen bars within walking distance of the one in which we were sitting.

And inside the bar in which these actors were seated there were at least a half-dozen barstools remaining *unoccupied*, any one of which I could have chosen to park myself and kill a few hours.

So why did I choose to walk into *that* particular bar on *that* particular day and take a seat on *that* particular barstool? I'll never know. I won't even speculate.

The man in civilian clothes announced that he was rotating back to the states in two weeks.

The man to his right asked the man in civilian clothes what was his "M.O.S." An M.O.S. is a "Military Occupational Skill," in other words, his job in the Army.

The man in civilian clothes said he was the "feature writer" for the *Stars and Stripes* daily newspaper. What was a "feature" writer I wondered.

"They are trying to find my replacement," said the man in civilian clothes. "But there aren't many newspaper writers around."

Time to grab that brass ring, I thought, not about to miss this golden opportunity!

"I couldn't help overhearing your conversation," I said. "But I wrote for my school newspaper in high school, and later for my campus newspaper while in college. Is there any way I could apply for the job as the feature writer?"

"I don't see why not," he answered. "Nobody else has applied for it. By the way, where are you stationed now?"

"My name's Al Provost," I said.

"And I'm Jon Powell. Pleased to meet you Al." We shook hands.

I explained that I had just arrived in Seoul to attend projectionist school for a week. Then I had to return to Camp Page to take over as the camp Audio-Visual guy. "But I'd much rather write for the newspaper. Can you help me?" Did Jon Powell catch the desperation in my voice? I was hoping he did.

"Let's have a beer, then we'll drive out to the newspaper office in Yungdung-po. We have plenty of room and you can spend the night. I'll drive you back to Seoul in the morning."

After finishing our beer and Coke we climbed into his Jeep and merged with the traffic heading south across the Han River Bridge. A "po" is a city district. After leaving the Yongsan district we crossed the Han River Bridge into Yungdung-po, a major residential area of Seoul. A few miles farther south Jon Powell turned left and parked in a walled-in residential property. Not a business operating anywhere in sight.

"Well, we're home," said Jon Powell as he parked beside a two-story red brick building alongside several other Jeeps, each of which had

STARS AND STRIPES painted in black letters on a white background just below the windshield.

"Is this where you work?" I asked curiously. We were standing smack-dab in the middle of a Korean residential area. Not a "round eye" (American) anywhere in sight.

"That's correct," said Jon Powell. "It's also where we live. The newspaper is located on the ground floor and we live and sleep on the second floor."

"I don't see any army barracks anywhere," I observed, walking to the edge of the property and peering left and right along the street. "Where do we eat?"

"Follow me," he said. We walked about forty yards to the street corner, where we turned left and stopped.

"This is the road to Osan," said Powell. "That's the largest military air base in Korea. Look to your right and you'll see about a hundred yards from here the cyclone fence and the guard post. That's where we take our meals."

"What's on that base?" I asked curiously, not expecting to see an army post in a residential district.

"That's Company A of the 502," said Powell.

"The 502 what?" I asked curiously.

"The 502 Military Intelligence Battalion," he said. "This is where the U.S. Army interrogates captured North Korean communist espionage agents," he explained.

"So we eat our meals with American prisoner interrogators?" I asked, my interest being whetted almost instantly. And then I thought: What in the world have I stumbled onto now? Could I ever hope to be so lucky? How utterly fascinating!

But first things first I thought. And the very first thing I had to do would be to land the job as the feature writer with the *Stars & Stripes* daily newspaper. Then I would wrangle a position as a Communist espionage agent interrogator. Eat your heart out, James Cagney! You too, Humphrey Bogart!

Intelligent young man that I was, I naturally assumed that as this particular interrogation center was ensconced smack-dab in a residential area and on a main, heavily-traveled road no less, then this likely was not the *main*, or *central* interrogation center.

However upon inquiry Jon Powell assured me that this was indeed the only communist interrogation center in Korea. Of which he was aware, he stated. I would investigate further, but the matter at hand was making certain I became Jon Powell's replacement *Stars & Stripes* feature writer.

We returned to the walled compound, found a parking space and went inside the two-story red brick warehouse that had been converted into a newspaper press room and living quarters for eight-to-ten members of the Korea Bureau of the *Pacific Stars & Stripes* daily newspaper.

The Interview

"Let's go see Sergeant Kelsey," said Jon Powell as he led me into an office in the corner of the pressroom. "Kelsey is our Bureau Chief," he added. The three of us sat at Kelsey's cluttered desk and Jon Powell began his sales pitch, accepting what I had told him earlier at face value because I was sincere and had an honest face. Or rather I suppose. And perhaps I would learn the role of this mysterious "feature" writer. At least it sounded more important than did a mere "reporter," that conjured images of "book reports" in Miss Mamie Baldwin's fifth grade.

Sergeant Kelsey began the conversation as though he had read my mind.

"So I'm going to interview you for the job as the feature writer," he said. "If you pass the test I'll explain what you'll be doing." He stood and walked to a table in the corner of the room. He returned and placed before me a newspaper written in English. It was a copy of *The Korea Times*, Seoul's major English-language daily.

Without comment the sergeant opened the newspaper. Scanning the pages he checked off five of the stories, then announced the test.

"Provost, this is your chance to realize a dream," he said. "If you pass this test I promise I'll have you working for us within a week or two. Are you ready?"

"I'll do my best," I said.

"Okay, I have checked five articles in the paper. Your job is to *rewrite* these articles, telling the same stories but using different words. In other words when I read the two articles I must get the impression that each is a different story. Take as much time as you need. We'll leave it with you. Good luck, son." As they stood to leave Jon Powell gave me a big smile and a *thumbs-up*.

So I picked up a writing pad and opened the newspaper to the first checked story. It wasn't easy. However I realized my fate should I fail. And I vowed failure was simply not an option. So the choice was not between the newspaper and being the Camp Page projectionist for the next year. Rather, the choice was between the newspaper and slashing my wrists with a rusty straight-razor while sitting naked in a bathtub.

When I completed the last article I put down my government-issued No. 2 yellow and glanced at the large clock on the wall. Only twenty-five minutes had passed.

Without second-guessing myself I walked to the door and opened it. Sergeant Kelsey looked up at me.

"Why are you sweating, Provost?" he said. "It couldn't be all that bad." He laughed. I didn't. Nor did Jon Powell.

The bureau chief sat at his desk. He picked up the newspaper and the writing pad, looking back and forth between the two stories. After he had read the third article and my rendition he placed both items on the table and extended his right hand to me. I shook his hand, uncertain of whether the handshake meant "Welcome to the *Stars & Stripes*," or "I'm sorry it didn't work out."

"I don't need to read anymore," he said. "I could not have done better myself. Welcome to the *Stars & Stripes*, son. You're now the new feature writer." Just like that.

"And now that I have the job," I said, "Maybe you could tell me what a feature writer is." So he told me. And I was as happy as a pig wallowing in mud.

"I'll telephone Col. Creel, the Eighth Army Information Officer, early tomorrow morning," said Sergeant Kelsey. "He'll cut you orders for transfer to the *Stars & Stripes*. You'll be here within a week or ten days."

"Provost came here from Camp Page to attend the projectionist course," said Jon Powell. "He begins the course this coming Monday, and it runs through Friday," he added.

"Okay Provost, go ahead to projectionist school this week and return to Camp Page. Just don't mention your *Stars & Stripes* assignment to anyone. I have a feeling the commanding officer of Camp Page isn't going to be pleased when he finds out he still doesn't have a projectionist."

"When should I expect to get my orders transferring me to Seoul," I asked eagerly while trying my best to remain calm.

"Probably by Thursday of next week," replied Sergeant Kelsey. "I'll get in touch with Col. Creel by phone the first thing Monday. Meanwhile just go through projectionist school. Telephone me here at the newspaper if you need me. And by the way, Provost, welcome to the *Stars & Stripes*." We shook hands and Jon Powell drove me back to the Eighth Army barracks in the Yongsan district of Seoul. We shook hands and I thanked him again.

"Al, my help is not entirely altruistic," he replied. "The feature writer is the main cog in this wheel called the *Stars & Stripes* daily, as you will soon learn. They were going to keep me in Korea until we found a replacement. So you see, you're helping me as much as I'm helping you. I still have to stay over for a few weeks to show you the ropes, which I'm glad to do."

Camp Coiner Projectionist School

The following Monday morning I rode the large olive drab army bus to Camp Coiner, a small army post that housed the Eighth U.S. Army Projectionist School. There were twenty students in the class, and from Monday to Friday we had an interesting time and became quite proficient in the operation of a half-dozen audio-visual (AV) machines.

The projectionist school was part of the 181st Signal Company, commanded by Captain Kenneth J. Offan. The course was taught by PFC Ralph D. Chapman.

The projectionist school provided quite capable instruction in seven types of projectors including two types of motion picture projectors, four slide projectors and one sound reproducer.

Before the course ended on Friday afternoon I had passed the practical test on each instrument and when we boarded the army bus for the ride to Seoul I had in my pocket my laminated license with my photo on it.

By Friday morning I had not received any word from Sergeant Kelsey concerning my re-assignment from the U.S. Fourth Missile Command to the *Stars & Stripes*. I telephoned the newspaper office in Yungdung-po and spoke to Sergeant Kelsey.

"I spoke with Col. Creel (Col. George Creel, Eighth Army Information Officer). He advised you to return to Chunchon on the Korean train tomorrow (Saturday). Your transfer and re-assignment orders will be 'twixed' (teletyped) to Camp Page Personnel on Monday. You'll be in Seoul by next Wednesday. Again, congratulations Provost."

I returned by Korean train to Camp Page on Saturday and walked from the train depot to Camp Page. After lunch I reported to the Audio-Visual Center located in a large building at one corner of the compound, in my hand clutching my bright-and-shiny laminated card attesting to my proficiency in the operation of those seven aforementioned Audio-Visual (AV) machines.

I walked into the building, greeted the AV supervisor and handed him my license. He was happy because I could take over and he could rotate stateside. Or so he believed.

Suddenly the telephone rang. The AV supervisor lifted the receiver.

"AV Center," he said. He listened intently.

"Yes sir, colonel," said the supervisor. He listened briefly. Then he spoke.

"Yes sir, colonel. Right away sir." He replaced the receiver and looked up at me.

"What's going on?" I asked innocently, as if I didn't have a clue.

"That's the base commander. He said he wants to see you in his office right away. He didn't sound very happy. What's going on?"

"Damned if I know," I lied. But of course I knew.

I trudged over to base HQ and checked in with the corporal seated behind the desk. Minutes later the door behind the desk opened and one really big red-faced senior Army officer spoke in an angry voice.

"Come on in, Provost. And explain yourself if that's possible."

I entered the colonel's office. He motioned me to sit at a desk. Without further prodding I explained in as brief a time as possible about meeting Jon Powell in the bar, learning of the newspaper's need for a feature writer and visiting the newspaper office.

"Well I hope you realize what a bind this puts me in, Provost. Now I'm going to have to keep my projectionist here for another few weeks while I send someone else to projectionist school. Your orders indicate that you are to report to the newspaper office on Wednesday, three days from now. But you just sit tight until I see if I can rescind those orders. I'll let you know. That's all soldier."

There were two ways to tell the colonel was not happy with my insolence. He failed to return my crisp military salute, and he called me *soldier* when he knew my name was *Provost*. *C'est la vie* in Camp Page in 1962.

However apparently in a difference of opinion the only person who could settle a disagreement between two bird colonels was the Commanding General of Eighth U.S. Army, in this case Major General Meloy.

And apparently General Meloy sided with the Eighth Army Information Officer, Col. George Creel, because two days later the colonel's aide telephoned the AV Center and told me to pick up my orders.

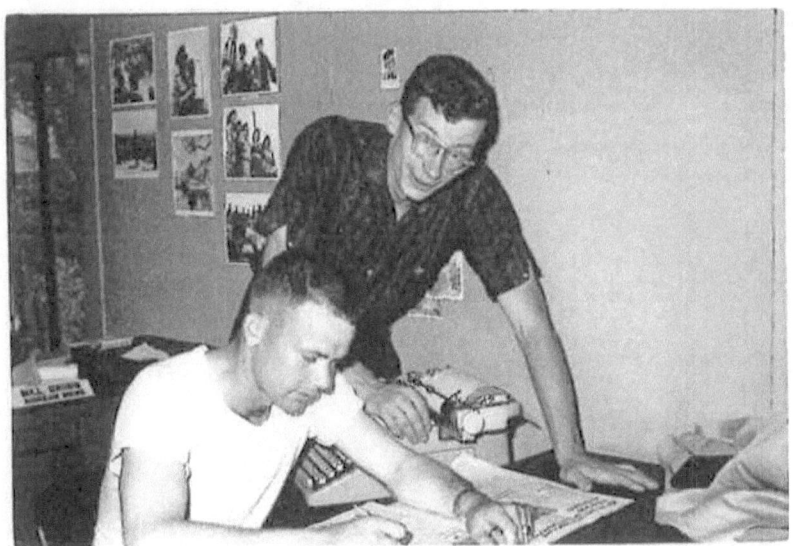

Stars & Stripes Press Room. March 1962. This photo was taken a few days after jon Powell had recruited me to replace him as the newspaper's Feature Writer. Jon believed in me and I owe him a lot.

Chapter 4

◇◇◇◇

A Most Interesting Life Begins

At 3:30 p.m. on a bleak, cold and drizzly April 3, 1962 I stepped off an unheated Korean passenger train in the Seoul Train Depot, where I was met by a reporter for the *Stars & Stripes*. One could readily spot those Jeeps by the wooden bar that rested at the base of the windshield, that read in black letters on a white background, *STARS AND STRIPES*. I had telephoned the small newspaper compound from Chunchon and informed Sergeant Kelsey of the train's arrival time in Seoul.

As we drove through the center of Seoul, once again I found myself in a sea of foreign-language, bronze-skinned people, and it still bothered me to no end that I couldn't understand most of what was spoken by any of the masses. Nor could I read anything printed on storefront or road signs. It was almost depressing.

One encouraging sign was that the so-called *writing* appeared to be in the form of simple block letters. Smart lad that I was at my young age, I had bet myself that I could learn the Korean alphabet and thus how to read the language in approximately ten-to-twelve hours. And I had.

Another thing that should help in learning the alphabet was that everything appeared to be *printed*; none of it *in cursive*. I had studied several languages, one of which was Russian. The printed Cyrillic was somewhat legible. However cursive Russian was like trying to read a different language.

Truth be told however, a foreigner attempting to learn printed English would likely confront a similar problem with cursive English. But first things first. I was about to embark upon a four-year adventure at the young age of twenty-two. Thinking back, I would not trade the experience for any amount of money.

On the half-hour drive from the Seoul Main Railway Station to the (relatively) small *Stars & Stripes* compound my fellow journalist-driver explained the operation of the *Stars & Stripes* as follows.

There were five regular reporters including Sergeant Kelsey, one feature writer (myself) and the commanding officer, a captain. Sergeant Kelsey actually served as the "bureau chief," in charge of handing out assignments to the other four regular reporters, who covered Seoul and its suburbs. These reporters returned to the compound at the end of the day.

"So what's the difference between the four daily reporters and the feature writer?" I asked, certain that a wee bit of apprehension was showing in my voice.

"You cover the rest of South Korea, which means you likely will be living on the road a good part of the time."

"Where will I stay at night?" I asked.

"If you can't make it back here by midnight, just stop at any military post. Tell them who you are and they will put you up in a transient barracks for the night, feed you supper and breakfast the following morning, and gas up your Jeep."

"What if I'm not near a U.S. Army base at midnight?"

"This occasionally happens. In that case just stop in at any Korean hotel for the night. Sergeant Kelsey will give you a fistful of "won" (Korean dollars) so you'll always have money on you. Although it's against Korean law for a Korean to possess U.S. money, Koreans still would rather be paid in American dollars."

"What's so magical about midnight?" I asked curiously.

"There's a midnight-to-6:00 a.m. curfew throughout South Korea. Sergeant Kelsey will give you an I.D. card, signed by Col. Creel. The front side is in English and the reverse side is in Korean. The I.D. card allows you to break the curfew, so if you drive through some small village at 2:00 a.m., a Korean cop or Korean Army M.P. may stop you. But just show him your U.N. Command I.D. card and he'll let you pass. It's never been a problem."

At this point in my introduction to the newspaper we had run out of time to learn before we had exhausted the subject matter. But the fellow reporter had been very helpful and I thanked him. And at the same time I asked him one last question:

"By the way, where do I get my stories?"

"You're the hotshot feature writer," he said. "Nobody tells you what to write. However if you write about what you like, most of your 37,500 readers will like these same stories."

"Why 37,500 readers?" I asked.

"Because there are 37,500 American troops in Korea. You should be thankful that you have a very large audience. Your name will be the by-line on every story you write, and after a few months of writing, every G.I. in Korea will know who you are." Sounded good to me anyway. An unknown one day. A household word the next. Who knows? A nobody one day – winner of the Pulitzer Prize the next!

"And by the way," said the reporter, "Your audience also includes the more than 5,000 American civilians who live and work in the greater Seoul area."

Meeting the "502" Prisoner Interrogators

At 5:15 p.m. we turned left off the busy street and parked inside the compound. I picked up my duffel bag from off the back seat of the Jeep and we went inside the two-story red brick building. The large press room took up most of the first floor, while the bathroom and bunk area occupied the second floor.

Jon Powell met us just inside the front door. "Good to see you Al," greeted Powell. "Toss your duffel bag on one of the bunks and we'll walk down and have supper with the guys at the "502."

The *Stars & Stripes* compound was situated about a hundred yards north of the road to Osan. A left turn would take you to Osan Air Force Base, about forty miles to the south. If you continued straight ahead on the Seoul-Yungdung-po road for thirty-five miles you would reach the port city (*town*, really) of Inchon.

In 1962 you couldn't turn right at that intersection. If you did you would crash into one of the best Chinese restaurants in Seoul. It was a dead-end to street traffic heading west.

At the three-way intersection Jon and I walked on the side of the road for about 150 yards until we came to a large walled-in area, the top of the white-painted cinder blocks containing barbed wire.

About midway down the wall heading east we came to a metal gate guard post, at which stood a U.S. Army M.P. armed with a Carbine rifle and a sidearm. The young M.P. and Jon Powell greeted one another, and Jon introduced the guard and me.

"Add Provost to your list of guys from the newspaper," said Powell. "Al will be with us for the next year or so."

The guard and I shook hands. Then he reached into a small guardhouse and withdrew a clipboard. He recorded my name, rank and serial number, beside which he wrote *STARS & STRIPES*. Then he wrote this same information on a wallet-sized card and handed it to me.

"Just show this card to the M.P. at the gate for the next week or so. Once everyone knows you on sight, they'll just wave you through."

From the gate we walked up a grassy slope to the large mess hall. We entered and found a couple of seats. The Korean waitresses were serving supper, and Jon introduced me to the other "502" G.I.s as they entered.

"You'll get to know these guys here at the prisoner interrogation compound as well as you'll know the *Stars & Stripes* reporters. Officially this army post is Company A, 502 Military Intelligence Battalion. We just call it the '502' or the 'interrogation center'!" He paused in thought, as though unsure of himself.

"I'll go ahead and caution you on this one matter, to get it out of the way," he said.

"And what is that?" I asked.

"Sergeant Kelsey will go over this with you later tonight but I'll touch on it now," he said.

"Everything on this compound is classified Top Secret. Therefore you won't see or hear anybody talking about prisoner interrogation. So if you want to ask any of the Americans anything just make sure it has nothing to do with what goes on here."

"I've got the message," I said. "Mum's the word. No talking shop."

"I'll go over the reason for this rule after we get back to the newspaper, where we can speak freely," said Jon.

"The mess hall here opens at 6:00 a.m., so you can walk over for breakfast anytime after that."

"If we have less than a dozen men at the newspaper, what time do we get up in the morning?" I asked. For the life of me I couldn't see a dozen men falling out at 6:00 a.m. in any sort of military formation.

"We're pretty laid-back around here," he replied. "Because we're reporters we can't keep a regular schedule. So if you don't make a habit of it, nobody's going to complain if you aren't out of your bunk by 7:00 or 8:00 in the morning."

Throughout supper I mentally compiled about three dozen questions I was dying to ask about the interrogation center, but following Jon Powell's admonition I used discretion and instead talked about my new life as a writer for the *Stars & Stripes*.

During supper I listened to the constant chatter of the Korean waitresses and busboys, renewing my vow to learn the Korean language as quickly as possible. Jon Powell appeared to be an intelligent lad, so I asked him whether any of the reporters were learning Korean, formally at least.

Jon said he (Powell) was the only one who had taken any Korean language courses that were offered at Eighth Army headquarters located in the Yongsan district in downtown Seoul.

"But I'll make it easy for you," he said, motioning one of the prisoner interrogators over to our table.

"Bill, this is Al Provost. He's my replacement as the feature writer. What's the quickest way for him to learn the language?"

"Well, before we come to Korea we have to undergo a year of language training at the Army Language School in Monterey, California. I still have all my language books and the wire recordings. If you're determined, I'll see if I can locate a wire recorder and get you started."

"I'd be glad to pay you for the use of your books and the recording tapes, Bill," I said eagerly.

"You all just sit tight," he said. "I'll be back in a jiff."

Fifteen minutes later Bill returned, carrying a medium-sized cardboard box. He placed it on the table, then withdrew several items and placed them on the table before me.

"I brought you the first five Korean language books from the course, plus a wire recorder and the recording tapes. These should get you started," he said.

"Thank you so much," I said. "How long can I keep these materials?"

"I'm rotating back stateside in seven months," he responded. "Let me have them by then. When you finish these first five books let me know and I'll get you the next five. Korean is a difficult language to learn but if you're dedicated you'll pick it up fast. Good luck to you."

As the prisoner interrogators and *Stars & Stripes* reporters drifted in, took seats in the dining room and ordered supper, I found it quite easy to tell one group from the other. The interrogators were the ones speaking Korean to the waitresses. I was impressed. And envious.

Looking around the dining room it became quite obvious to me that for some odd reason all the G.I.s seemed to be in a good mood. Puzzled, I mentioned this to Jon Powell.

"You're pretty darned observant Al," he said. "I guess it has to do with liking what they do. I like my job at the newspaper. Nobody crowds us and we have a lot of latitude in what we write about and freedom as to when we come and go. And neither the reporters nor the interrogators ever have to carry a weapon or fall out in formation."

"No wonder everyone's in such a good mood," I said.

"In addition the prisoner interrogators receive a double pro-pay in their pay envelope."

"What's a *double pro-pay?*" I asked.

"Some jobs require a knowledge your run-of-the-mill G.I. does not possess. One of these is speaking a foreign language, in this case Korean. A second specialty is the interrogation of espionage agents. This is an art within itself. Both these specialties require special training. The army recognizes this and pays you well for these specialties. Pro-pay stands for *proficiency pay.*"

"Do newspaper reporters receive pro-pay?"

"No. However over and above their base pay each month, the prisoner interrogators receive one pro-pay of $300 for being a Korean linguist and a second pro-pay of $300 for being a prisoner interrogator. This comes to extra pay over and above their base pay. It's $600 per month total or $7,200 per year." Certainly impressed me, it did.

Chapter 5

◇◇◇◇

The Luckiest G.I. in Korea

When we arrived back at the office Sergeant Kelsey was seated at his desk. He motioned us to sit across from him, then tossed a notepad and pencil to me.

"There's a lot to learn about your duties, so feel free to take notes." I picked up the pad and pencil, moving the items closer to me.

"Stop by Eighth Army headquarters as soon as possible. Introduce yourself to Col. George Creel, head of the Eighth Army Information Office. Col. Creel is your real boss. He'll give you a laminated I.D. card that has your photo on it."

"When do I use the card?" I asked.

"The front side is in English, the reverse side is in Korean. It identifies you as a *Stars & Stripes* reporter. It allows you to travel on the roads during the 12:00 midnight to 6:00 a.m. curfew and it allows you to travel by car, truck, boat or airplane anywhere in Korea. If you should have any problems – which you won't – just telephone me here at the bureau or Col. Creel at Eighth Army headquarters.

"What is it you want me to write about specifically?"

"That's the beauty of your job," put in Jon Powell. "Write about what interests you and nine times out of ten it will be of interest to your audience, that includes not only the 37,500 G.I.s stationed in the country but about 5,000 civilians living in the Seoul area."

"You'll have a Jeep permanently assigned to you," said Sergeant Kelsey. "You can gas it up at any military post in the country, and there is a full five-gallon gas can in your Jeep. Just keep it filled and you'll never run out of gas."

"Do I need to be back here by any certain time?" I asked.

"You certainly don't," responded Kelsey. "If it's late it's safest to stop in at any military post rather than try to drive at night. Every base has transient barracks. Just show the M.P. at the main gate your I.D. card. They'll find you a bunk, a shower and something to eat. Just gas up your Jeep before you get on the road the following morning." I couldn't wait to get started.

"If you really get stuck in bad weather, you can always stop in at a Korean hotel and spend the night. The Korean police will look after your Jeep," said Jon Powell.

The Military Armistice Commission (MAC) Meetings

"In addition to writing about what you find interesting, there are a few mandatory events you must cover," said Sergeant Kelsey. "The most important are the *MAC* meetings."

"What's a *MAC* meeting?" I asked quizzically.

"*MAC* stands for Military Armistice Commission," explained Kelsey.

"As you may know, following the end of the fighting, there was no peace treaty signed, only an Armistice. So technically, the north and the south are still at war."

"So do the two sides meet every few months?" I asked.

"Not exactly. If one side does something to offend the other, the offended party will call for a meeting at the JSA, or *Joint Security Area*, which is located in Panmunjom, about a ninety-minute drive north of Seoul. We'll let you know when a meeting will be held. Just leave in your Jeep early that morning in plenty of time to get there before the meeting starts. You need a special pass to enter the JSA."

"How will I know what the meeting is all about?"

"Just stand outside the large Quonset hut where the meeting is being held. You'll hear the American officer read off the complaint."

"Once I get to the JSA is there someone who can fill me in on what's going on?"

"Yes. Locate Captain Cecil Neely. He's the highest ranking M.P. He'll fill you in on what's going on. And bear in mind that all our M.P.s are armed, as are the communist North Korean and communist Chinese guards. Other than these precautions treat the story as you would any other story. Just stay on your toes. These gooks are nuts."

Even after all these years I still recall thinking: Thanks a lot, Sergeant. First you tell me I will be rubbing elbows with three dozen or so fully-armed, trigger-happy communist guards for several hours, then in the same breath you expect me to treat this story the same as I would treat *any other story*? Really? And then you tell me they're *nuts*?

The plan I formed in my puerile young mind was to locate Captain Neely as soon as I arrived in the JSA, and not allow him out of my sight until it came time to floor the gas pedal in my trusty Jeep and scratch gravel leaving the area, heading south to safety.

The Dictator's Press Conference

"A second mandatory story you and I must cover is General Park's upcoming press conference at the Seoul National Palace," said Sergeant Kelsey.

"What's the occasion, and who exactly is this General Park?" I asked.

"About a year ago General Park took over the South Korean government in a coup, and has been a dictator ever since. This will be his first major press conference. You are going to interview him and I'm going along as your driver. I'll help you come up with eight or ten good, meaningful questions."

This newspaper gig was getting more complicated as it went along. First I was going to be trapped in a small place called the *Joint Security Area* with three dozen or so armed-to-the-teeth, American-despising communist guards.

And should I survive this experience I could look forward to being trapped inside a building called the *Seoul National Palace* with an equally despised Korean dictator.

Fleetingly I considered getting into my (own personal) Jeep, driving it down to the Central Rail Depot in downtown Seoul, abandoning the vehicle, taking the first train to Chunchon and begging the Commandant of the Fourth Missile Command to take me back.

Eager to get started on my new career as a photojournalist, I had a few ideas already. Not only that, I knew exactly how to get to the location of these two stories, namely Chunchon, home of the Fourth Missile Command – and the colonel who hated my guts – and projectionist school from where I had just graduated. I passed these thoughts by bureau chief Sergeant Kelsey and he was impressed.

"Looks like you are ready to go," he said. "Contact the commanding officer of each of these outfits. Tell him you want to write the story and agree on a day and time to drive up. Make sure you arrive on time. And one more thing."

"Which is?" I asked expectantly.

"When you report to the base commandant be certain you take a few photos of him at his desk and out in the field. You are then applying the first rule of military journalism, that is everyone, from the lowly enlisted Private to the three-star general, wants the folks back home in Podunk, Iowa to see him commanding troops in Korea. Do you get what I mean?" asked Sergeant Kelsey.

"I'll welcome this and any advice you wish to offer," I said.

The "Stringer" and the Single Lens Reflex

"Later on I'll tell you how to earn more money as a *stringer* than you get in your pay envelope each month," said Jon Powell. "And it's all quite legal," he added.

"You may as well go ahead and tell him" said Sergeant Kelsey. "Make it worth his while."

"Okay, here goes," said Jon Powell. "How may G.I.s work at the projectionist school?" he queried.

"I'd say about six or seven," I said.

"Okay, when you write the story take enough photos of each soldier that depicts him in a *supervisory* role, regardless of his rank."

"Do I just have the film developed down at the Main PX at Eighth Army headquarters in Yongsan?" I asked.

"That's the easy way to do it. This is the reason each of us carries two cameras – one for the *Stars & Stripes*, the other for ourselves," said Powell.

"Anyway, ask each soldier where he's from and which newspaper serves his hometown. The G.I.'s relatives can get you the name and address of the newspaper. When you send a copy of the personalized story to his hometown paper, include with it a copy of the article that appeared in the *Stars & Stripes*."

"I'm certain there is a good reason for doing this," I said. "But what is this reason?"

"Authenticity, in a nutshell," said Powell. "The *Stars & Stripes* is trusted worldwide. The editor of the hometown newspaper knows he doesn't have to double-check the facts of your story because the bureau chief, Sergeant Kelsey, has already determined that the facts are accurate."

"Sounds reasonable to me," I said. "By the way, how much should I expect to be paid for each story?"

"Newspapers and often magazines usually pay what they refer to as *scale*, which is so many dollars for each linear inch of print, no more and no less," said Powell. "It averages out at about $50 per story."

"How will I receive payment?"

"Go down to the main U.S. Post Office at Yongsan. Rent a post office box. Newspapers will pay you by check. Set up a bank account with the Bank of America, also located at Yongsan. How much you earn as a *stringer*, or *freelance reporter*, is limited only by how hard you're willing to work."

"We need to set you up with at least three cameras," said Kelsey. "Can you take your own photos?"

"I'm a pretty good photographer," I said. Or lied. "But what if I wasn't?"

"We have a Korean that we use as a photographer and interpreter. He works for us full time. His name is Kim Ki Sam."

"Let's do it this way, if it's all right with you Sergeant Kelsey. You told me already that there are usually a few Koreans in each town or village who speak at least rudimentary English?"

"This is true," said the Sergeant.

"So I think I'll pass on Kim Ki Sam, for the time being anyway. I'm going to begin studying Korean on my own, and within a month or six weeks I'll be able to find my way around. What kind of cameras do you have?"

"We use mainly Nikon 35mm and the *single lens reflex*."

"I've heard of the single lens reflex. What about it?"

"It's a more expensive but a better quality camera. But whereas you hold the 35mm up close to your eye to take the photo, you have to hold the single lens reflex down about waist-high and center the object in the square frame."

"Like aiming through a Norden bombsight?"

"You might use that analogy. It definitely takes more practice getting the object lined up to take the picture but it gives you a better quality photo, especially when the subject is a person."

"Well let me practice on the single lens reflex and on my first assignment I'll try it out. And still let me have the two Nikons also."

"And remember to take plenty of film with you," advised Sergeant Kelsey. "You might think you're going to just write one story, but when you get there you see where you can do one or two more stories."

And By the Way, About Those Korean Roads...

"We're going to get you fixed up with your cameras and your Jeep tonight," said Kelsey, opening his desk drawer and withdrawing two road maps of South Korea. He tossed them onto the desk in front of me.

"Don't let these out of your sight," cautioned Kelsey. "The Koreans know even less than do you about map-making. These two maps are from Eighth Army Transportation, but you may even spot a few errors on those maps." Really? (I said to myself.)

"May as well tell Al about the condition of the roads so he'll know what to expect," added Jon Powell in a serious tone.

"Okay, here's an interesting statistic," said Powell. "Only about five percent of the roads in South Korea are paved, and this five percent are mainly roads in towns," he added, allowing this fact to sink in.

"For example Chunchon is the capital of Kangwon Province. The two times you went from Seoul to Chunchon you traveled by Korean train, did you not?"

"This is correct."

"When you go to write your story about Camp Page and the Honest John Rocket, you'll travel by Jeep. Your three-hour drive from the city limits of Seoul to the city limits of Chunchon is made solely on dirt roads. Not even any gravel."

"Sounds downright dangerous to me," I said.

"You bet it is. Up in the steep hills the dirt roads are carved into the side of the mountains. Don't hesitate to cancel a visit to Kangwon Province if the weather report on AFKN (Armed Forces Korean Network) calls for rain or snow on the day you plan your trip. Be extremely careful."

"What's the reason for so few paved roads, or should I try for an educated guess?"

"You would be correct," said Powell. "This is 1962. The Armistice was signed in July 1953, only eight or nine years ago. The nation is just too darned poor to afford to pave more roads."

Better to Have it and Not Need It...

As I sat at Sergeant Kelsey's desk discussing my travel plans with the bureau chief and reporter Jon Powell, I realized I was about to embark upon the adventure of a lifetime. Following breakfast with the prisoner interrogators down the street at the mess hall inside the "502" prisoner interrogation compound, I would climb into my *own personal* Jeep with my maps of South Korea and head north crossing the very wide and deep Han River linking Yungdung-po with the Yongsan district of Central Seoul.

Inside the Eighth U.S. Army headquarters I would locate the building that housed the Eighth Army Information Office and Col. George Creel. The colonel would issue to me an I.D. card for use anywhere in Korea, essentially identifying me as a Press Representative of the United Nations Command and warning anyone who reads the card not to interfere with me in the furtherance of my mission.

With the magical *Open Sesame* I.D. card I could begin in earnest my job as a fledgling *Stars & Stripes* reporter.

However something was missing here.

What was missing was the inescapable fact that I was going to begin driving around Korea, unable to speak or read much of this (very) foreign language, and I would be expected to do this without being armed with any kind of weapon.

My loving parents raised seven children. If any of the seven turned out to be stupid, I was not one of these. I had already been informed by one of the Americans that because we were not a combat unit, we were not cleared to carry sidearms.

But what about carrying a *concealed* weapon? So I put the question to the American in the form of a hypothetical. First however I asked the outgoing feature writer the reason none of the reporters carried a weapon.

"Mainly because the four daily news reporters never leave the Seoul area. In fact at least two of them just hang out at the Eighth Army Information Office down at Yongsan and write about goings-on of a military nature. So these reporters are never likely to need a weapon for protection."

This made a lot of sense. Now I could not be so bold as to ask an American whether *he himself* carried a concealed weapon in his travels alone through the Korean countryside. However I did learn that he took a young Korean male about 40 years old along with him for use as a translator and photographer when he left the Seoul area to research and write.

"I've already told Sergeant Kelsey that I won't need the Korean's help," I said. "I'm a pretty good photographer on my own, and I plan to begin studying Korean at night."

"Okay Provost, now you're painting a different picture. If I were going out on my own I believe I would carry a concealed weapon, but not a Model 1911 .45 cal. Automatic."

"And the reason?"

"Simply because it's illegal for a Korean to possess an American military weapon."

"So how do I get a non-military weapon?"

"Let me telephone a Korean friend of mind at his home. He'll be able to advise you about buying a weapon." We telephoned the Korean and I introduced myself and told him what I needed.

About an hour later I heard the front door open and in walked a smiling Korean about forty or so years old. He was carrying a cloth-covered box that, if I had to venture a guess, would contain an American-made handgun.

I took the box from him, carried it into the dormitory and shoved it beneath my pillow. A few minutes of small talk ensued after which the Korean departed, carrying with him my heartfelt thanks.

During the fifteen months I served as the feature writer for the *Stars & Stripes* I carried the cloth-wrapped weapon and extra shells (the box was too bulky) hidden beneath the driver's seat in my Jeep. I never once left Seoul without it, and fortunately never had to use it. Better to have it and not need it, than to need it and not have it. Always good advice.

The Secret of the TDY Orders

Each of the reporters carried three proofs of identification; a driver's license, a United Nations Command I.D. card, identifying us as reporters and admonishing everyone not to interfere with us in the furtherance of our duties, and a *TDY sheet* that listed each of the nine members of the *Stars & Stripes* unit, giving our name, rank and level of security clearance if the reporter possessed such clearance.

The driver's license and the United Nations I.D. Card contained a photo of the person. For obvious reasons the TDY sheet did not contain photos.

New TDY Orders – TDY stands for *Temporary Duty* – were issued every sixty days, copies were made and each man carried a folded copy with him whenever he left the *Stars & Stripes* compound, as a form of identification.

We *Stars & Stripes* reporters undoubtedly had the most enviable jobs in Korea. With these three means of identification we could literally go anywhere at anytime of the day or night, and as long as what we were doing did not violate any laws we were about as untouchable as a G.I. in Korea could be.

The first TDY Orders on which I was included came out about ten days after I arrived at the compound. When the copies were handed out I had not been in the office.

So when I drove into the compound, parked the Jeep and walked into the press room, Sergeant Kelsey the bureau chief asked me in a joking manner why I was so special.

"What do you mean?" I said, not having seen a copy of the TDY Orders.

Kelsey handed me a copy and immediately a small circle formed, everyone wanting to know the meaning of the Orders.

And sure enough, two of the reporters had no security clearance, four had Secret Security Clearances, and even the unit commander, a captain, had only a Secret Security Clearance. And sure as shootin' there was my name and rank, followed by *Top Secret Security Clearance*.

Now I knew that the Top Secret Clearance could only have been given by the FBI when I applied for a job there, or else by the FBI when I applied to attend OCS at the time I joined the army.

But I wasn't about to tell this to these clowns. Nosiree. I thought quickly.

"Well, if I told you the reason I hold a Top Secret Security Clearance, I would be violating my security clearance because telling you the reason I *hold* the clearance cannot be done without telling you what's *in* the clearance. I hope you understand, but keep in mind that I came here from the Fourth Missile Command, which is the home of the Honest John Rocket."

The older, higher ranking enlisted men were somewhat put out because the *lowest-ranking* reporter not only was the hotshot feature writer but in addition possessed the highest security clearance.

However the one who took my having a Top Secret Clearance hardest was the *Stars & Stripes* commander, a captain by rank. It appeared to be beyond his comprehension as well as a personal slight that a lowly Specialist Fourth Class newspaper reporter could hold a Top Secret Security Clearance when he, a captain, held but a Secret Security Clearance.

See Special Orders Number 72, dated 25 March 1963, a year after I arrived at the Stars & Stripes compound on April 3, 1962.

Therefore when I signed the letter indicating that I declined to attend OCS, the army had to assign me to my next post. And the army does this in a logical manner.

A review of my personnel record, known as a DD Form-214, showed that I possessed a college degree in Physics-Mathematics, and that I had undergone the eight-week course in Advanced Artillery Training in the operation of the 105mm Howitzer at Ft. Sill, Oklahoma in the fall of 1961.

So the army was searching for a military post at which my skills were needed, and they came up, quite logically, with the U.S. Fourth Missile

Command located in Chunchon, the capital of Kangwon Province, way the hell up in the boonies of northeast South Korea.

The only thing wrong with the army's decision to ship myself and a thousand other seasick G.I.s on a 28-day voyage across the Pacific was that nobody cared to know how I felt about the matter.

It was getting to be late in the day and the reporters were busy typing up their stories in preparation to "twixing" the materials to Tokyo's large bureau, where the newspaper was printed. By 3:00 a.m. more than 40,000 copies of the paper had been loaded aboard the gutted KC-135 Tanker plane for the early-morning delivery to Kimpo Air Base south of Seoul and from there distributed overland to dozens of U.S. military bases throughout South Korea.

The *Stars & Stripes* was a big operation, and the army was determined to keep its soldiers informed of the outside world.

The Coveted TDY Orders

Enclosed is a copy of Special Orders Number 72, dated 25 March 1963 and issued by Headquarters Special Troops, Eighth United States Army. I had been assigned to the *Stars & Stripes* nearly a full year, having arrived from the U.S. Fourth Missile Command at Camp Page on April 10, 1962.

New Special Orders were issued every sixty days. Each man was given a copy of the Orders, that he carried with him when he left the compound. *TDY* stood for Temporary Duty.

As the Order shows, there were only eight men assigned to the *Stars & Stripes*. The Commanding Officer, Lieutenant Sala, possessed a *Secret* Security Clearance. The highest ranking enlisted man, Master Sergeant Marshall, grade E7, and I were the only men in the eight-man unit who possessed a Top Secret Security Clearance. I was not related to Norman Provost; this was merely a coincidence.

By necessity the Orders were open-ended, stating simply: *TDY to: To points in Korea deemed necessary*, and the *Purpose* of the Orders was *Stars & Stripes Activities*. As one can readily see, there was a lot of freedom packed into Special Orders Number 72.

HEADQUARTERS SPECIAL TROOPS
EIGHTH UNITED STATES ARMY
APO 301, SAN FRANCISCO, CALIFORNIA

SPECIAL ORDERS   25 March 1963
NUMBER   72   E X T R A C T

10. TC 201. Indiv pl on TDY as indic. UCMR parent orgn. TDN.

USA Elm Pac Stars & Stripes (5765) APO 301
~~SARA, GARY C~~   ~~2D LT INF   Scty clnc Secret~~
MARSHALL, WILLIAM E   MSGT E7 Scty clnc Top Secret
GREENOUGH, WILSON C   SFC E6   Scty clnc Secret
KELSAY, WARREN A   SSGT E6 Scty clnc Secret
PROVOST, NORMAN J   SP5 E5   Scty clnc Secret
PROVOST, ALTON L   SP4 E4   Scty clnc Top Secret
NEWLAND, LYNN C   PFC E3   Scty clnc None
PUTTERMAN, MICHAEL S   PFC E3   Scty clnc Secret

TDY to: To points in Korea deemed nec
WP date: 5 Apr 63
Pd: Approx 60 days
Scty clnc: As indic
Purpose: Stars & Stripes Actv
Auth: EUSA Cir 310-10
Acct clas: NA
Sp instr: Tvl by govt auto mil acft and ry dir. Tvl perf under this
          O const dy contem by para 4250.3 JTR. Govt rats and qtrs will
          be prov for pds of tvl and TDY dir by this O.

Special Order No. 72

Chapter 6

◇◇◇◇

The Bridge that Wasn't There
Or
What Happened to My Bridge?

If you were to tell me you had no phobias, I would counter that you were being downright disingenuous. As long as memory serves me I have been saddled with several phobias, among these being a fear of enclosed spaces and a fear of bridges, high or low, whether made of wood, metal or concrete. Also large bodies of water including any river, ocean, sea, inlet or tributary more than five feet wide and eighteen inches deep. It doesn't take much for me to break out in a cold sweat and my intestines to turn to mush.

The great-granddaddy of all my phobias however – prolonged drum roll here – is of course a fear of *heights*. I become downright sweaty and get weak in the knees the instant my foot touches the third rung from the bottom of a ladder. I'm strictly a two-rung kind of guy. It pays to know your limitations. Personal security is having both feet – at the same time moreover – planted on dry land, preferably in the Sahara.

During my two tours of duty in Korea, the first as the feature writer for the *Stars & Stripes* daily and the second as a prisoner interrogator and Korean linguist, the Honest John Rocket was the state of the art (though of questionable accuracy) surface-to-surface missile.

Following eight weeks of Basic Infantry Training in the stifling heat of July and August of 1961 I was posted to Ft. Sill, Oklahoma for eight weeks of Advanced Artillery Training. With an undergraduate degree in Physics-Mathematics I understood well the Principles of Trajectory of missiles, rockets and artillery shells large and small.

For this reason I was assigned to the U.S. Fourth Missile Command in Chunchon within two weeks of opting out of Officer Candidate School in December 1961.

One day in mid-April 1962 I received a telephone call from Col. Creel, my boss at the Eighth Army Information office inside Yongsan compound in Seoul. He asked me to stop by as soon as possible. He had an assignment for me that he did not wish to discuss over the telephone. Sounded downright intriguing, it did.

Seemed as though the U.S. Army recently had developed a new missile, the specifications of which Col. Creel either did not know, or knew but decided to leave this conversation to the Brigadier General commanding the army base southeast of Seoul.

I stopped by Col. Creel's office the following morning. He gave me the name of the one-star commanding general of the base I was to visit the following afternoon. Be there at 1:00 p.m., said Col. Creel. As I moved to the door on my way out of his office he picked up two maps from his desk and handed them to me.

"This is a special assignment, Provost. Report back to me when you return and before you write the story."

And before I could ask the colonel why he was being so dadblamed secretive about the assignment, he shooed me out the door. A man of few words was Col. George Creel.

When I arrived back at the small (relatively-speaking, that is) *Stars & Stripes* compound, I placed one of the maps on the corner of my bunk, and stuffed the other inside the canvas satchel where I stored my three cameras and cache of film.

Col. Creel had told me the one-star's name, the name of the military post and the name of the Korean town closest to the military post.

Author's note: I have elected to leave some names, ranks, military installations and weapons unnamed. It was either that or make up a bunch of fictitious names, which required extra effort and added nothing to the story. Col. Creel and Sergeant Kelsey are real persons.

Col. Creel informed me that my appointment with the Brigadier General was for 1:00 p.m. the following day and told me the road I should take to reach my destination.

After breakfast the following morning down the street at the "502" mess hall I returned to the *Stars & Stripes* office. Assuming (without reason) that Col. Creel had given me two maps in case I should lose one of them, I left one map on the corner of my bunk, and placed the second map inside my canvas satchel, grabbed my wrapped .38 cal. chrome-plated revolver and headed for my Jeep, assuming that the two maps were identical, which upon a cursory glance certainly appeared to be the case.

The day was sunny; it was mid-April and the weather was pleasant. About two hours out I stopped in a village to get what in 1962 Korea was the equivalent of a Kool-aid colored drink, then continued on my way.

I had consulted the map given to me by Col. Creel. It depicted a very long bridge over a godawful wide river. The bridge must have been at least a quarter-mile long. I said a little prayer that it would not be constructed of wood.

Driving farther on I spotted the river a good two miles before I reached it. As I rounded a bend in the road my heart skipped a beat. It was monstrous, brown with mud, with a slow current. Unnerving, it was.

I observed at water's edge two Korean vehicles, a lorrie and a passenger car. What I didn't see anywhere however was a *bridge*. I turned to the lorrie driver.

"Bridge?" The question required but one word, inflected.

"No bridge. Only pole man," he responded.

"What is *pole man*?" I asked querulously, I'm certain with the accompanying blank expression on my face.

In response he pointed out to the middle of the massive body of water where if I squinted my eyes I could barely make out a vehicle sitting on what appeared to be a flimsy raft, with several men standing around the vehicle. Again I turned to the driver of the lorrie, who appeared willing to help.

"No bridge?" I asked almost pleadingly.

"Sorry, no bridge," he responded, now shaking his head to stress the finality of his answer.

Suddenly I thought to show him my map given to me by Col. Creel. I spread the map out on the bed of the lorrie. It definitely showed a long bridge spanning the river at that point.

The man lifted the map and turned it over several times, inspecting it closely.

"This old *Japanese* map," he said.

"You need other map," he added apologetically.

I took the map, held it up and read the Legend at the bottom.

> Prepared by the Army Map Service, Corps of Engineers, U.S. Army, Washington, D.C. Compiled in 1956 from: Japan Road Map, Army Map Service Sheet 3, edition 1946, Sheet 4, edition 1950 (reliability good). Users noting errors or omissions on this map are urged to mark hereon and forward directly to Commanding Officer, Army Map Service, Washington, D.C.

So much for *errors or omission*, I thought. Damn. My (Japanese) map included both. Probably lots of both, if truth be told.

This revelation was a shock to my senses. So what I was holding in my sweaty palms as I gazed in apprehension at this ungodly expanse of muddy water was a *Japanese* road map printed in 1946, the year following the Japanese surrender in August 1945, ending World War II.

But not to worry, the U.S. Army Map Service had stated that the "reliability" was "good."

As I stood at the water's edge – but not too close, mind you – I considered my rather limited options.

As I was standing there I peered downstream. Consulting the map, I pointed to the Korean town (village really) close to the army base that was my destination. I would never make my appointment with the general if I backtracked and drove south to the next bridge, that the driver of the Korean lorrie stated *did* exist.

It was apparent that rather than lose credibility – which is about all a newsman has to offer – I would have to overcome my fear of large bodies of water. At least for the moment anyway.

Suddenly I observed as the small raft loomed on the horizon of muddy water. Apparently the raft had deposited the vehicle on the opposite bank of what I could only characterize as a *menacing* body of muddy water that would be difficult to refer to as a "stream" because it was barely moving. I quickly dubbed it *Lake Mud*.

I was comforted – though not much – by two things. First of all the small "pole barge," as the Koreans called the wooden raft, had apparently deposited the vehicle safely on the opposite shore and was returning for its next customer.

Second, the Korean lorrie was twice as large as my Jeep, and if the lorrie driver was willing to trust this large vehicle to a ride on the pole barge, then my comparatively much smaller Jeep should be able to make it safely across. I prayed.

Both the driver of the lorrie and the driver of the automobile waved for me to go ahead of them. I thanked them and turned to the pole barge worker who appeared to be in charge.

"How much?"

"Hundred won," he responded.

A *won* is a unit of Korean currency. One hundred won equals one U.S. dollar. So the three Koreans were going to charge me what amounted to one U.S. dollar to *pole* my Jeep across Lake Mud to the opposite shore.

Even though I was placing my safety – and possibly my life – in the hands of these three Koreans, I was determined to capture the moment on film. But we made it, with me holding my breath most of the way. And as you can see in the photos, the Jeep was never secured in any way to the pole barge. Nor would be the lorrie next in line at water's edge.

When I had driven my Jeep off onto dry land I gave the man 900 won ($9.00) rather than the $1.00. No way in hell would I take this "water route" on my return trip.

However the three *pole bargers* had been helpful, and I arrived at the army base on time. Upon my return to Seoul I made three copies of the photos and put them into my canvas satchel. Several months later I passed by the area again and gave the photos to the pole bargers. They were, in a word, simply ecstatic.

Still however I never took another "Voyage of Terror" on that river. Nosiree.

The Story I Did Not Write – The Nike Battery

When I arrived at the base I reported to the office of the Commanding General. I saluted him sharply, then we shook hands.

"This is a relatively small base, as bases go," he began. "However we are strategically located to test a new weapon because we need a lot of open range to do this. We're in no hurry, and following our meeting it will be too late for you to return to Seoul tonight. We'll put you up in the officer billets for the night just to ensure your research material will be safe." The general explained the situation as follows:

The Honest John Rocket is a surface-to-surface missile. Its range is 15.4 miles more or less, depending on the payload. By comparison the range of a 105mm Howitzer shell is but 7.0 miles.

An Honest John Rocket payload can be either conventional or nuclear. However an artillery shell from one of the *larger* Howitzers can reach nearly 15.4 miles, the range of the Honest John. Thus when dealing with conventional weapons a large artillery shell will suffice; the Honest John Rocket would be considered a redundancy in this situation, based on my knowledge of missiles.

Therefore as of 1962 anyway, any warhead associated with the Honest John Rocket would necessarily be nuclear in nature. Without bringing it up in conversation then, both the Brigadier General and I knew the purpose of my trip had nothing to do with the Honest John Rocket nor with any of its cousins.

I had been given this assignment because of three reasons. First, I was the only reporter with a knowledge of the subject matter, that is, artillery, rockets and missiles. Second, I was the only reporter who possessed a Top Secret Security Clearance. And third, I was the only reporter who understood the language of nuclear weapons.

Therefore my best educated guess before the one-star uttered a word was that the U.S. Army was about to test an advanced surface-to-surface, long-range missile powerful enough to reach North Korea carrying a *tactical atomic warhead*. Had to be.

But it wasn't. Not even close.

"Before we discuss the reason you're here Provost, we need to show you the newest weapon and explain its operation. Come with me."

In his Jeep we drove across the base to the far side of a small building, where we were met by a colonel, a captain and several sergeants. No introductions were made.

"Okay captain," said the general. "Deploy when ready." The captain gave a hand signal to one of the sergeants and the side of the small building opened up. A horizontal platform rolled out and stopped about twenty feet from the building. Resting on the platform were six sleek white-painted missiles each about ten feet long and two feet in diameter.

Again without further commands the captain pushed a single large black button located on a control box and as the six missiles elevated I silently counted one thousand one, one thousand two, etc.

I heard six identical metal clicks as the missiles locked in the *Ready* position.

"How many, Provost?" asked the general.

"I counted seventeen sir," I responded.

"You're close, Provost. It took only *sixteen* seconds to ready the six missiles. I'll go over the specifications later this afternoon. Of course we're talking in terms of surface-to-air missiles," said the general.

"Then we're planning for these missiles to destroy an equal number of North Korean or Chinese jet aircraft?" I asked presumptively.

"With one main caveat," he interjected.

"This is certainly a state-of-the-art weapon. However we haven't yet found our accuracy nose-to-nose to be any greater than thirty percent. We did find that by employing a *shotgun* approach our kill rate rose to greater than seventy percent when used against Chinese heavy bombers."

"Therefore the weapon guidance system must be set to deploy at a close enough range that the enemy plane would have no time to evade the barrage of more than likely thousands of razor-sharp titanium projectiles," I speculated.

"You're quite correct in your assessment of the situation, Provost," he said. "As we both know, all it would take would be a half-dozen metal shards to enter the nose intake of an approaching jet and the plane would not be able to remain airborne."

"General, may I ask a question that might appear premature?"

"Go right ahead Provost."

"Why do you need me, sir? Can't I just write the story and turn it in to my bureau chief?"

"No Provost, because of the nine men in your *Stars and Stripes* unit, only you and the Master Sergeant have a Top Secret Security Clearance.

Even the captain commanding your unit does not have a Top Secret Clearance. Furthermore the Master Sergeant who does have a Top Secret Clearance is not a reporter."

"I understand, sir."

"So the reason you are here is to do your research and write the story. But don't type it. When you have finished it, take your handwritten story to Col. Creel. I'm the one who has asked that the story be published, but others will decide this."

"What are the odds of publication?" I asked.

"We'll give the success rate, stating that it can destroy any enemy aircraft before it reaches South Korea. Because it is a conventional weapon, I believe the odds are three-to-one that we can get the story printed."

I recall thinking at that exact moment that the first time the new surface-to-air missile *should* come to light should be the first time a squadron of Chinese long-range bombers crossed the DMZ. No way in hell would I give the North Koreans advance warning.

The last two hours of the day were spent in the general's office. He gave me chapter and verse on his pride and joy, even allowing me to photograph the six-missile battery in the raised and locked position, but from a distance of thirty feet. Seemed fair enough to me.

I informed the general that with all the technical information at my fingertips, I could write the story in less than an hour, and he could have input. He agreed. An hour later I had quoted "a high-ranking officer" several times, and both our names should have been in the byline.

After breakfast in the officers' mess hall the following morning, the general had the motor pool service my Jeep. I took several photographs of him seated at his desk, he gave me directions back to Seoul, we shook hands and I departed. Though not in the direction of Lake Mud. No way in hell!

When I reached Seoul I drove directly to Eighth Army Headquarters in Yongsan and reported to Col. Creel. I gave him my handwritten story. He read it carefully, nodding in agreement as he went along.

"Good job Provost," he said. "I'll be in touch."

About ten days later I returned to the *Stars & Stripes* compound from an assignment, to see a note on the small bulletin board that Col. Creel would like to hear from me. I telephoned him immediately.

"Your story went all the way to G-2 (Army Intelligence) in Washington, D.C.," said the colonel. Everyone liked the story. However for the immediate future the *brass* (highest ranking officers) have decided to shelve it. But you did a good job."

"Thanks for informing me, colonel," I said. "By the way did you give the general the bad news?"

"Yes, and he was disappointed, as you might imagine. But he'll get over it."

At the time I wrote *The Story That Was Never Printed* I was a Specialist Fourth Class, known also as a *Spec-4*, in rank about the same as a corporal. But I still had an opinion based on my knowledge of rockets, missiles and weaponry. After giving the situation a lot of thought, I agreed with G-2. I would not have printed the story because doing so would have served no useful purpose.

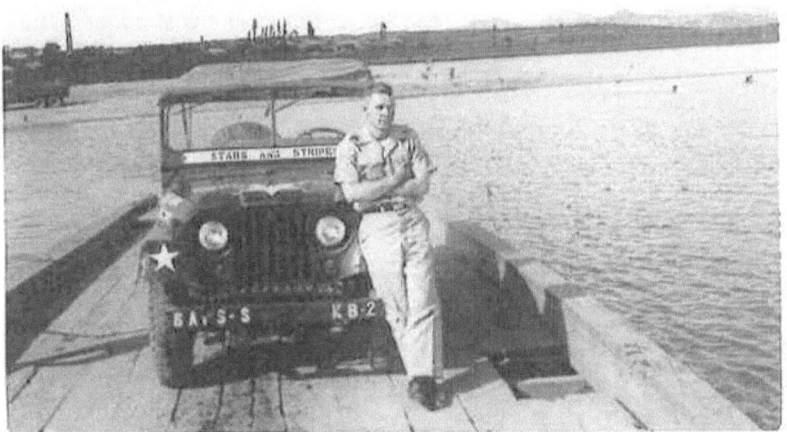

April 1962. Crossing the wide Han River with my Jeep, on a "pole barge," powered by three Korean pole-bargers. The map given to me by Bureau Chief Sergeant Warren Kelsey, showed a long wooden bridge. However it turned out that the road map was a postwar Japanese map, dated 1946, the year following Japan's defeat that ended World War II

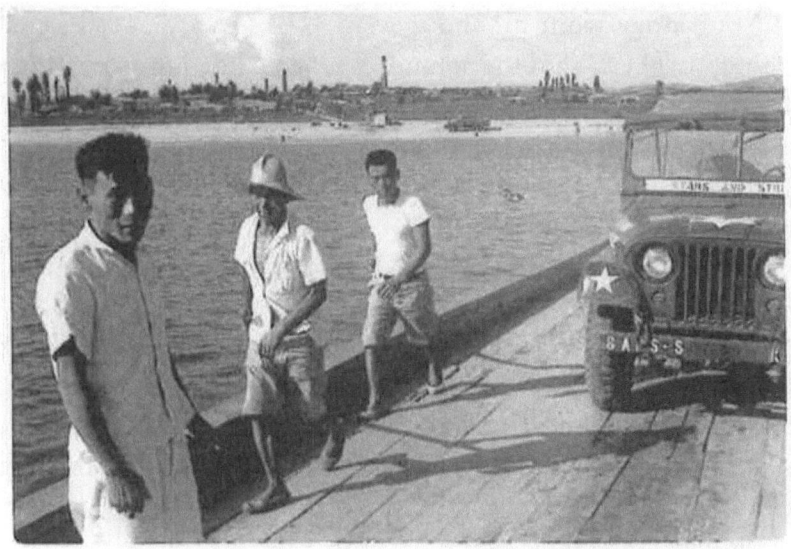

April 1962. Three Korean "pole-bargers" ferrying my Jeep and me across the wide Han River. For this trip they charged me the grand sum of one U.S. dollar. Instead I paid them nine U.S. dollars. They were ecstatic..

Chapter 7

◇◇◇◇

The Korean Dictator's Press Conference
My Frightening Near-death Experience

On May 15, 1961 I graduated from Berry College, located near Rome, Georgia, with a degree in Physics-Mathematics.

The following day, May 16, 1961, Kim Jong Pil, a young Lieutenant Colonel in the South Korean Army, and his uncle-by-marriage, Major General Park Chung Hee, seized the South Korean government in a lightning but relatively quiet coup.

A year later, in mid-April 1962 I experienced my terrifying encounter on Lake Mud, the rickety pole barge and the bridge that wasn't. And a month later my nerves were slowly recovering from that trauma when one day Sergeant Kelsey approached my desk while I was typing a story for the newspaper.

"Provost, do you recall when you first came aboard my telling you about the anniversary of General Park's coup?"

"Yes I do recall," said I. "Should I do a story in honor of the historic occasion?"

"Even better than that," said Kelsey. "We have been invited to take part in a press conference on the anniversary, along with reporters from the Associated Press, United Press International, the Korean language daily *Tong-a Ilbo* and the English language daily, *The Korea Times*. So you'll be rubbing elbows with some pretty good journalists and probably will be on TV."

"Are you coming along also?" I asked.

"Yes, as usual I'll come along as your driver, and I'll sit with you at the interview," said the sergeant.

We were informed by Col. Creel's office of the date, place and time of the event. General Park's aide informed us the general was setting aside time in his busy schedule for the interview, which would give us time to ask perhaps four or five questions. These questions were to be submitted to General Park's office three days prior to the date of the interview, and of course the general would select which questions could be asked. Given the circumstances of the times, the process appeared reasonable to me, as yet I numbered but a few dictators on my Christmas card list, and longed for more.

Because the other reporters were all civilians, I asked Sergeant Kelsey whether we should wear civilian clothes so as not to stand out like a couple of sore (khaki-clad) thumbs. But after giving my question the customary serious thought it deserved, Kelsey voted for us to wear our uniforms because it made the U.S. Army appear more professional. I went along because one, it made no difference to me one way or the other and two, Kelsey had about three stripes more than I had on my sleeves.

And Sergeant Kelsey's decision to wear our uniforms may well have saved my life. We'll never know for certain.

I believe the interview was scheduled for noon on May 17, 1962 in the conference room inside the Seoul National Palace in downtown Seoul. Sergeant Kelsey was driving his Jeep and I was riding shotgun, holding on my lap a folder containing the list of six questions we would be allowed to ask.

The general's aide instructed the reporters to walk from the entrance lobby down a long hall to the conference room and that General Park and his four bodyguards would follow shortly. I took this as a silent acquiescence that if I had my single lens reflex ready I would be able to get a nice close-up of the dictator marching down the hall.

In preparation for taking the photo I held the single lens reflex down at waist-level and opened the case. When I heard heavy footfalls behind me I moved to the side, prepared to take my Pulitzer Prize-winning shot.

Timing was everything. I had to click the shutter hoping that General Park would enter the picture from my right literally at the exact instant I clicked the shutter. I would have only one chance to frame the general in the center of the picture; however I was confident in my photography skills. However,…

The instant I clicked the shutter everyone within ten feet of the camera heard the sharp *Click*! And when they turned toward the sound all they saw was a U.S. Army soldier holding a metal object down in front of him at waist level, then aiming it.

In that instant of time two of the four bodyguards, apparently believing a shot had been fired from the "gun" I held in my hands, grabbed my upper arms and slammed me up against the wall as the other two bodyguards hustled the general down the hall and into the safety of the conference room.

At the same time, one of the two bodyguards snatched the single lens reflex from my hands, breaking the strap. Suddenly I understood. These goons thought the camera was either a bomb or a weapon. All they heard had been a sharp *Click*! from an object I was holding down in front of me at waist level.

"Camera. Camera. Camera!" I shouted, releasing my grip on the camera and raising my hands in the universal "Don't shoot – I give up" stance.

At the time I took my photograph there had been a Korean photographer standing on the opposite side of the hall filming the event with a movie camera. See Photograph.

When I shouted "Camera. Camera. Camera," while pointing to my single lens reflex down at my waist, one of the bodyguards shouted "No. *That* camera!" and pointed to the movie camera up in front of his face, and his movie camera did not produce a sharp *Click*!

The bodyguard, knowing nothing about single lens reflex cameras, assumed that if it were indeed a camera, it would be held up to the eye, not down at the waist.

I asked the bodyguard to return my camera. Stupid request.

"No. After," he said. He apparently was telling me that I could have my camera back after the press conference. In fact he did not return the camera until Sergeant Kelsey and I were in our Jeep leaving the parking lot of the Seoul National Palace. And he still wasn't smiling.

I don't believe Sergeant Kelsey and I fully appreciated what had occurred that day in the hallway of Seoul National Palace until later that night. However the story was told in that single photograph.

As I suspected I had timed the shot perfectly. Two bodyguards led the pint-sized dictator walking from right to left. I had not wanted the four bodyguards in the picture, and they had not been.

And I had to time the shot such that although I was standing perfectly still, when I clicked the shutter General Park, moving at a brisk pace, would be centered near the middle of the picture. And when we developed the film the dictator was just where I had planned for him to be – near the center of the picture.

Thus at the exact moment the shutter made the sharp *CLICK*! my camera was no more than three or four feet from General Park and his four (two in front and two behind) no-nonsense bodyguards, and out of respect for the general no one standing in the hallway had been talking.

Everything had occurred in the heat of the moment and later, on our fifteenth review of the events, we agreed that had I been wearing civilian clothes and not my uniform I might have been taken for an assassin and shot dead by the bodyguards.

Over the course of fifteen months as a photojournalist I must have taken several thousand photographs, dozens of which today, more than fifty years later still elicit fond memories. Many of the photographs are stories within the story, for example the story of Lake Mud, The Pole Bargers and The Missing Bridge.

Still today one of my all-time favorite stories within a story is my escape by the skin of my teeth in the hallway of Seoul National Palace. And I still shudder to think of what the outcome of the story might have been.

In addition the only photograph taken on the roll of film had been the one taken of General Park in the hallway of Seoul National Palace. This was in keeping with a hard and fast rule of journalism: Never put photos of more than one story on one roll of film. The reasoning should be obvious. Editors will hate you. Forever.

And General Park appeared in the photo exactly where I intended – just entering the picture from the right. Impeccable timing, if I do say so myself.

A Deadly Twist of Irony

On May 16, 1961 General Park took over the South Korean government in a coup. Brilliant gambit it was. Simply brilliant.

A year later, on May 17, 1962 I interviewed the dictator inside Seoul National Palace. And nearly lost my life for my trouble. Until the end of my tour fifteen months later I never again entered Seoul National Palace. (Come to think of it I was never *invited* to return.)

Ironically, this hallway inside Seoul National Palace played an important and tragic role in the history of South Korea.

In 1972 General Park assumed complete dictatorial powers. Seven years later, in 1979 the dictator was assassinated by his bodyguards.

As he was marching down the hallway inside Seoul National Palace...

My experience the day of my interview with General Park Chung Hee is still quite vivid in my mind. Even today the shutter closing on my single lens reflex when I snap a photo makes the same sound as does the firing pin striking the base of a bullet when a shooter pulls the trigger on a revolver. Exactly the same sound. It's unnerving.

The Single Lens Reflex Camera

At Berry College (1957-1961) a classmate introduced me to a *single lens reflex* camera, and it quickly became my camera of choice. However I discovered that although its optics were superior to most 35mm cameras, it did have a few limitations.

One of these drawbacks appeared to be inconsequential. This was the sharp *Click*! When you snapped the photograph. A sharper and louder sound than that produced by the standard 35mm, you certainly were not going to sneak up on your subject while taking his or her photograph using the single lens reflex.

The second drawback of the superior-quality single lens reflex was the fact that the square-shaped viewfinder had to be viewed looking down from above, whereas the 35mm could be aimed from about any position because the camera was brought close to the eye when taking a photograph. Therefore the single lens reflex had to be held down at the waist while the photographer moved the viewfinder around in order to frame the subject. It was similar to a bombardier lining up his target in a bombsight.

Chapter 8

◊◊◊◊

Confrontation Inside the Joint Security Area

On the day Sergeant Kelsey "hired" me as the new feature writer, replacing Jon Powell who was on his way stateside at the end of his tour, I had a serious meeting with Powell and Kelsey, the subject of which was safety, specifically my own *personal* safety.

"First off, we don't have a choice of whether to cover the Military Armistice Commission (MAC) meetings, that are held inside the Joint Security Area (JSA) at the request of either the communist Chinese or the North Koreans, or the United States as a member of the United Nations Command," began the Bureau Chief.

"How much notice will I get before the day of the meeting?" I asked. "I don't want to be doing a story in Pusan (the southernmost port city on the Korean peninsula) and not be able to get back in time for the meeting."

"Don't worry, you'll have at least a week's notice," replied Kelsey. "I'll give you directions to the JSA in Panmunjom."

"Can I just drive my Jeep into the JSA?" I asked.

"That's not a problem for you because you have an official reason to be there. After all you're the hotshot journalist."

"How do I get my pass?"

"First just so you know, no peace treaty was ever signed ending the Korean War, only an Armistice. The JSA is not a tourist attraction, so you won't see many civilians there. At the main gate the M.P.s will give you a yellow pass with your name typed on it. The pass is valid only for the one day you are there."

"Where do I go to write my story?"

"Provost, in your entire life you will never be standing in as strange a place as the JSA in Panmunjom. First of all there is an equal number of communist Chinese and North Korean guards as there are American

M.P.s. Second, every one of these communist guards and American M.P.s is armed to the teeth, and all of them are just itching for a fight."

"How many in all?"

"There's gotta be at least seventy," said Jon Powell smiling. "Still wanna go, Provost?"

"What are my chances of driving out of the JSA alive?" I asked tongue-in-cheek.

"I'd say about 95 percent if you take certain standard precautions," said Kelsey.

"Okay, then I'll go. But what precautions should I follow, just in case?"

"Stay within viewing distance of Captain Cecil Neely. He's in charge of the U.S. Army M.P.s. If he gives you the *high sign* just calmly walk toward him. In addition don't walk *toward* any armed Chinese or North Korean. They're easily spooked. And don't raise your voice, and please don't laugh at *anything*. They'll think you're making fun of them."

"My last stupid question," I said. "Just in case someone does start shooting, what should I do?"

"Hit the ground and cover your head," said Kelsey. "If you try to run you become a large moving target. So just stay down until it's over, which won't take but a few seconds."

"When you take your first trip to the JSA, check to see how the communist guards are dressed. They wear these heavy woolen ankle-length coats. It's hard enough to walk in them and nigh onto impossible to run without tripping. They'd be sitting ducks."

"Thanks for your advice. Is there a place where I can write my story?"

"Yes," said Jon Powell. "The meeting is held in a Quonset hut. You can stand outside the hut and observe what is going on inside. Or you can sit inside the adjacent Quonset hut and listen to the meeting through the speakers attached to the wall."

"Just so you know Al, nine out of ten meetings are called by the Chinese and North Koreans. They use the meetings to harass the U.S. and the South Koreans, and as a propaganda tool," said Kelsey.

And it didn't take long. A month following all this good advice Jon Powell had returned to the states. I was busy learning the difficult language and attempting to memorize a map of South Korea, careful not to let the U.S. Army Map Service sneak into my gray canvas satchel a 1942 Japan road map, or worse.

One morning as I was typing a story Sergeant Kelsey poked his head out through the doorway of his office.

"Provost, your time has come to shine," he announced. "Leave for Panmunjom four days from today, early in the morning, say around 8:00 a.m. You should arrive at the JSA around 10:00 a.m., where Captain Neely will be waiting for you. And don't forget the precautions Powell and I gave you about how to survive the experience. Anything you need before you go?"

"Yes sarge," said I. "How about a bulletproof vest, extra thick, a fully-loaded Model 1911 Colt .45 and an M1 rifle with extra 8-round clips, for starters."

"Provost, a serious word about this story. You're a good writer. Bear in mind that high-ranking officers read the *Stars & Stripes* daily, and leave it up to you to keep them informed of what goes on at the MAC meetings. So be complete and feel free to add your own analysis to the facts as you see them."

A few months after beginning my travels through Korea I learned of the respect afforded to the *Stars & Stripes*. The paper contained all the news and sports as did any big-city daily, plus the stories written by the *Stars & Stripes* reporters including myself. The newspaper was printed in Tokyo and each morning at around 3:00 a gutted KC-135 tanker plane took off from Tokyo laden with crates of bundled newspapers bound for Kimpo Air Base south of Seoul.

Each of the newspaper's Jeeps sported a horizontal wooden bar resting atop the hood at the base of the windshield, that in black letters printed on a white background read STARS AND STRIPES.

Because the first thing the reader noticed when reading an article was the *byline*, just as the reporter told me when he met me at the Seoul Main Rail Depot upon my arrival in Seoul, it wasn't but a few months before it seemed that everyone knew me. Before very long I believed I knew the reason for this.

It had to do with my being the feature writer. The other four reporters simply wrote about the facts, that much of the time made for pretty dull reading, as these stories were written *by* soldiers *for* soldiers and offered no commentary.

The job of the feature writer however was to seek out the unusual stories that more often than not sought an analysis and opinion. For this reason the feature writer could speculate freely and quote the subject of the story extensively. I was good at both.

If I were on assignment and realized I could not make it back to Seoul before nightfall, I would locate the closest U.S. Army post. After showing the guards at the front gate my ID, which was the United Nations laminated card that contained my photo and signature, the guards would have me sign the guest register, then give me directions to the dining hall, transient barracks and the EM (Enlisted Men's) Club.

My jackets and shirts each contained two hand-sewn cloth nametags. The top tag, sewn in white letters, read simply *PROVOST*. The bottom tag, sewn with red thread, read *STARS AND STRIPES*.

The top tag conformed to U.S. Army dress code. The bottom tag was designed to have persons we met know we were from the *STARS & STRIPES* without us having to inform anyone of this fact.

So if I walked into an EM Club and took a seat on a barstool, before five minutes passed everyone sitting at the bar would know they had a reporter in their midst. Some conversations led to feature articles in the newspaper, while others I worked into articles written for the stateside hometown newspaper that would pay me a minimum of $50 in a check from the hometown paper.

On the morning of the scheduled Armistice Commission meeting inside the JSA at Panmunjom, I departed Seoul thirty minutes earlier than originally planned just to ensure I could make it to the meeting by 10:00 a.m. I admit to being a wee bit nervous.

Because of the international importance of the MAC meetings nearly (but not all) of the road from Seoul to Panmunjom was paved.

As noted previously, while I parked my assigned Jeep beside the *Stars & Stripes* building at night, as soon as I left the following morning, I removed my wrapped .38 Special, with shells, from beneath my bunk and hid it under the driver's side seat of my Jeep.

And lo and behold it wasn't until I arrived at the JSA that morning that I realized my unforgiveable error. There I was, sitting in my Jeep at the main gate, directly beneath the large sign that admonished:

NO WEAPONS ALLOWED BEYOND THIS POINT

Damn! No, double damn!

I was third in line to be allowed entry to the JSA. I was holding my magic Yellow Pass in my left hand, ready to hand it to the American M.P. standing at the guardhouse.

I quickly surmised that the only possible way out of this (damned) mess was to bluff my way through. I say this because I couldn't check my .38 cal. Smith & Wesson at the guardhouse. I was in trouble anyway because I was not even authorized to possess any weapon, military or civilian. I was about to commit a court-martial offense!

When came my turn I gave the M.P. my Yellow Pass. He glanced at my name.

"Provost. You're Jon Powell's replacement?"

"Yes sir, this is correct," I responded.

"You can park your Jeep anywhere on that grassy area," he said pointing to the neatly-trimmed lawn nearby. "I'll let Captain Neely know you're here."

Now that was easy. I just hoped he would not notice the sweat of fear beading on my upper lip. Who knows. Maybe I would live to bungle something else another day. I had once more dodged another bullet. I hoped.

As I parked the Jeep I observed a tall man walk out of one of the Quonset huts and approach the Jeep. I climbed out of the Jeep and gave the captain a crisp salute which he returned in kind.

"Good to see you Provost. I suppose you're Jon Powell's replacement?"

"Yes sir, and I'll try to do a good job for you and the other M.P.s."

"I'm sure you will Provost. Come with me and I'll show you around."

We walked over to a Quonset hut where workers, some Korean and others American, were setting up a long table with microphones.

"Do you see that white cord running down the middle of the table?" asked the captain as we peered through an open window at the side of the building.

"Anyway that cord is the dividing line between North Korea and South Korea. You can stand where we are standing now and listen to the entire meeting, that should last about an hour, or you can sit at a table inside the Quonset hut next door and listen in on the loudspeaker attached to the wall."

The JSA is a one-half mile diameter circular neutral zone straddling the Military Demarcation Line (MDL). The conference "room" is actually inside a Quonset hut.

The MAC conference room is so situated that the communist side of the table is actually located in North Korea and the United Nations negotiators are in the South Korean half of the Demilitarized Zone (DMZ). In 1962 U.S. Air Force Major General Joseph E. Gill was the senior officer representing the UNC/MAC.

Inside the JSA each side is authorized to have 35 armed guards. Standing in the midst of 70 armed soldiers, half of them communists, was disconcerting to put it mildly.

Upon seeing what I could only describe as an armed camp, I automatically added this to my ever-expanding list of phobias, that now included any half-mile diameter circle in which stood 35 communist soldiers armed to the teeth, while glaring menacingly – at me.

"I don't want to get in anyone's way Captain Neely. So what's your best advice?"

"First of all don't move around a lot, and don't make any *sudden* moves. The Chinese and North Korean guards are easily spooked. Stay close enough to me or one of my men. If you hear yelling or the sound of gunfire, hit the ground and cover your head with your arms. Don't ever run. Whatever the trouble is, it won't last a minute. That's a promise. Don't you worry Provost. Just write your story. We'll take care of you." But he neglected to add "That's a promise."

I took Captain Neely's advice. When the meeting began I stood outside the Quonset hut and peered inside, listening to the Chinese and North Korean negotiators spouting their venom.

After all this had been going on for awhile I walked to my Jeep, turned around, then leaned against it and began observing the communist Chinese and North Korean guards.

It appeared to me that the communist guards would rather be somewhere else than where they were. They just would not remain still, shifting their weight on one foot and then the other, their gaze darting back and forth.

All this was still a shock to the system. There were a total of seventy guards in all. And to think each of them was armed to the teeth while a stupid 22-year-old newspaper reporter was "armed" only with a No. 2 Yellow pencil was both unnerving and downright surreal.

As the hours passed I began to rethink my feelings concerning the S&W revolver resting under the front seat of my Jeep. I had from the beginning entertained doubts about being in the JSA among 35 communist guards armed to the teeth and I being defenseless.

But now I had two things on my side; a loaded .38 cal. revolver plus ten spare shells, and the key to my Jeep in my pocket. I was a Marksman's shot and felt that now I at least stood a chance in a firefight. That is, if I could get to my Jeep.

When it was time for me to depart on my return trip to Seoul, I went to say farewell to Captain Neely.

"Well how did I do, captain?"

"You did well Provost. You stayed out of our way, you didn't start any *Gunfight at the O.K. Corral*, so we made it safely through another MAC meeting."

"See you next time captain."

"You too Provost. Take care of yourself."

We traded crisp salutes and I was on the road south again. Relieved I'm sure.

The MAC meetings are proof that an act considered dangerous per se can, under the right set of circumstances become almost mundane. During the fifteen months I served as the feature writer for the *Stars & Stripes*, I attended about an equal number of Military Armistice Commission meetings.

However as routine as the situation might appear, still the intrepid newspaper feature writer must be prepared with his trusty camera to record any situation that might arise. One never can tell…

Over the course of so many months in which I attended so many MAC meetings I came to know both the Chinese communist and North Korean guards as well as the American M.P.s. From a distance.

One particular observation I made over the course of several months, one I never mentioned to Captain Neely, was that on more than a few occasions a certain American M.P. sergeant appeared to get closer to the Chinese and North Korean guards than seemed prudent. He would do this while never looking directly at them. They could never read his intentions because they couldn't make eye contact.

A common admonition of gun owners, that over the years has devolved into a paternoster of sorts, is as follows:

Never draw your weapon if you don't intend to use it. The M.P.s explained to me that they never made eye contact with the communists. Rather they kept their eyes on the communist guards' *hands*. Simply placing the guard's hand on his weapon triggered a deadly response on the part of the American M.P.s, which is the reason Captain Neely said that any firefight wouldn't last a minute.

Later on in this story I will present situations, backed up by photographs and the actual newspaper articles, that led our Bureau Chief, Sergeant Kelsey, to remark that I was a good feature writer because I had a "nose for the news." The altercation inside the JSA involving Captain Neely and his counterpart the North Korean officer, was one in which I was caught smackdab in the middle of the action. Definitely too close for comfort, and for weeks thereafter I cringed when I realized just how close I had come to death.

Becoming Part of the Story – Again

I arrived at the *Stars & Stripes* compound on April 3, 1962. As of December 25, 1962 I had attended at least ten of the negotiations. Every word spoken during these sessions was translated into Chinese, Korean and English and I had just about had it up to the proverbial "here" with the constant droning on of the communist negotiators' harangues.

When I tired of the official goings-on I turned my attention to observing the communist guards who milled around the JSA in small groups, no doubt for security.

The M.P. sergeant was still surreptitiously getting uncomfortably close to the North Korean guards. And I just knew it wouldn't be long before this M.P. sergeant exacted *payback* on some unfortunate North Korean guard. And just why was I so certain of this fact? Simply because I was so all-fired insightful, that's why. A thinker par excellence.

According to Captain Neely, in early December 1962, the day before a MAC meeting was held, a communist guard slapped a United Nations Command guard – not American – on duty in the JSA. A stinging blow, I was told.

So putting the old two and two together I reckoned that one of the communist guards was going to suffer payback, and the M.P. most likely to do the honors was the eager M.P. I had been watching for months.

And I had been spot-on in my prediction. On the morning of the day in question I arrived early at the JSA, where I was met by Captain Neely, who informed me of the communist guard's assault on the United Nations Command guard, British as I can best recall.

I did not mention my observations of the American M.P.; however I decided to stick to Neely like he was the *Tar Baby*, so I located him and did just that.

I was no farther than eight feet from the captain when *it* occurred. *It* happened so fast that I could have sworn the American M.P. must have practiced his moves beforehand.

When I looked up the American M.P. was stalking the hapless communist guard, and was quickly closing the distance. As he passed by the communist guard he landed a sharp right elbow to the guard's kidney, then moved away quickly, passing by me and positioning himself to the right of and behind Captain Neely, at the same time the communist guard yelped and spewed forth a string of profanities.

The guard's startled cries summoned the North Korean officer, and I heard the assaulted guard continue his string of expletives which were peppered with the slur *kae sikkya* (son of a bitch) as he pointed to the American guard.

His cries brought the North Korean officer, the assaulted North Korean guard and two other North Korean guards over to where I stood to the captain's left, and the American guard positioned himself directly behind Neely. I could have sworn he was laughing. I certainly wasn't. Laughing, that is.

As the four incensed communist guards approached us Captain Neely said under his breath, "Take your best shot Provost." I took two steps back, raised my 35mm Nikon and clicked one of my best photos of the year. When I started to take another photo the captain said, "That's enough Provost. Now get out of the way." Which I did. Quickly.

As Captain Neely stared down the four Koreans, six American M.P.s approached and stood to Neely's left where I had been standing.

Neither Captain Neely nor his M.P.s said a word. None of the Americans spoke Korean. And none of the communists spoke English, not even the North Korean officer.

So for several moments Captain Neely and the North Korean officer engaged in a "staring" contest. I distinctly recall looking at the weapon on each man's hip, worried as to who would draw first.

Fortunately however nobody reached for his weapon. Finally the North Korean officer angrily waved his hand in the air and the North Korean guards left the scene, not glancing back.

After the North Koreans had dispersed, showering us with insults, Captain Neely turned to me.

"Sorry about that Provost, but I didn't want you to get caught in the middle of a firefight. Did you get to take that one shot?"

"I understand captain. But I did get the shot you let me take and I think you'll like it."

And he did. However for at least a little while I lamented the fact that I never had a chance to film *The Gunfight Inside the Joint Security Area*. Oh, well…

Two photos are indicative of the unnerving incident. The photo from the *Stars & Stripes* shows the position of the players the instant I snapped the photo. This is the one shot Captain Neely allowed me.

The caption beneath the photo reads:
> In an incident reflecting the tension at Panmunjom, Korea, scene of Military Armistice Commission meetings, U.S. Army Capt. Cecil N. Neely eyes communist guards who had gathered menacingly around an unidentified U.S. guard (far right). The communist in the center claimed the American guard bumped him. The Reds dispursed after Neely stepped in the way and other American guards gathered around.

The Nikon 35mm photo was taken by Sergeant Kelsey. I'm on the left, Captain Neely is on the right and a U.S. Navy petty officer is in the center. The captain is explaining what the "altercation" was all about. Once again the intrepid *Stars & Stripes* reporter had become part of the story. And had survived.

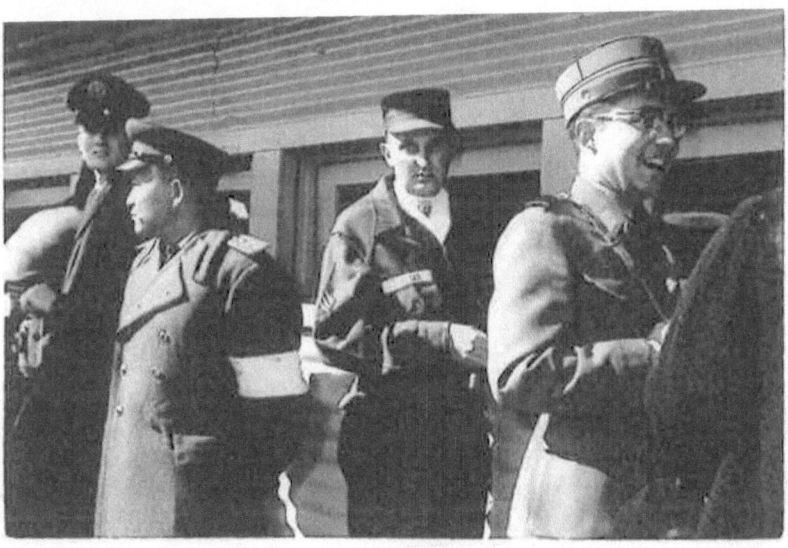

Panmunjom 1962. The Stars & Stripes Bureau Chief Sergeant Warren Kelsey, is shown standing between a North Korean army office and a polish army officer while negotiations are going on inside the Quonset hut just behind them.

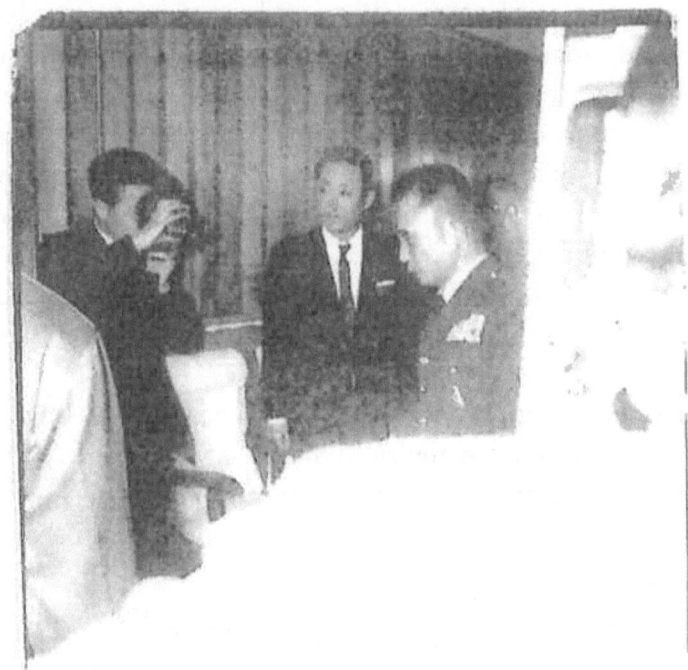

Summer 1962. General (read that "Dictator") Chung Hee Park's Press Conference that was held inside Seoul National Palace. I had to time the photo such that the general's four bodyguards - two walking in front of him and two behind - were not in the photo. I Itad time for only this one try because the bodyguards and General Park were in a hurry to get to the conference room.

(This photo and caption follow p. 97)
Place this photo after Chapter 7.
For caption of photo, see Chapter 7.
("The Korean Dictator's Press Conference")
Seoul National Palace, Summer of 1962.

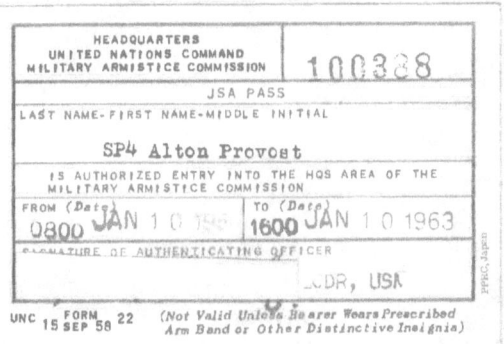

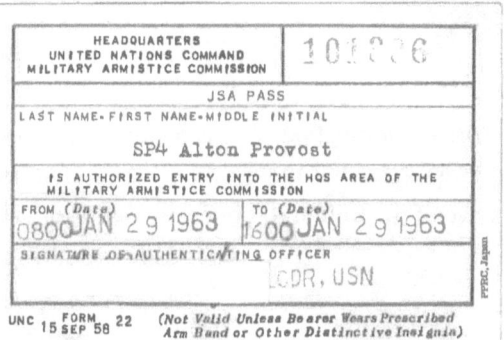

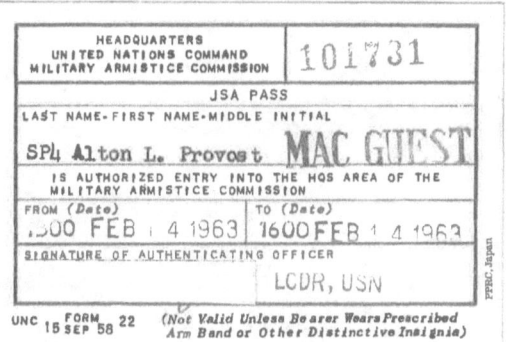

Panmunjom, February 14, 1963. What everyone just called the "Yellow-Pass," that anyone had to possess in order to be admitted to the headquarters area of the Military Armistice Commission, was valid only for the date printed on the card. During my 15-month tour of duty at the Stars & Stripes, I attended and reported on 14 such meetings.

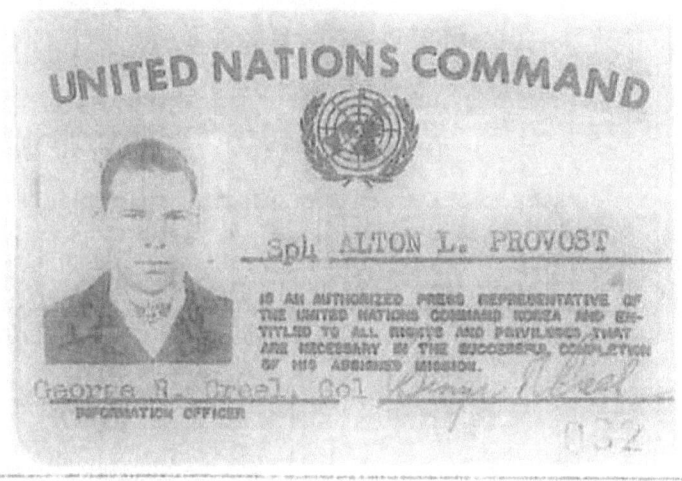

Seoul, Korea. Spring 1962. This is a copy of my United Nations Command Press Pass that identified me as an "Authorized Press Representative of the United Nations Command Korea."

```
                    HEADQUARTERS SPECIAL TROOPS
                     EIGHTH UNITED STATES ARMY
                    APO 301, SAN FRANCISCO, CALIFORNIA

SPECIAL ORDERS                                           25 March 1963
NUMBER    72                    E X T R A C T

     10.  TC 201.  Indiv pl on TDY as indic.  UCMR parent orgn.  TDN.

USA Elm Pac Stars & Stripes (5765) APO 301
   SALM,    GARY C              CD IN INF  Scty clnc Secret
   MARSHALL, WILLIAM E                     MSGT E7  Scty clnc Top Secret
   GREENOUGH, WILSON C                     SFC E6   Scty clnc Secret
   KELSAY,   WARREN A                      SSGT E6  Scty clnc Secret
   PROVOST,  NORMAN J                      SP5 E5   Scty clnc Secret
   PROVOST,  ALTON L                       SP4 E4   Scty clnc Top Secret
   NEWLAND,  LYNN C                        PFC E3   Scty clnc None
   PUTTERMAN, MICHAEL S                    PFC E3   Scty clnc Secret

   TDY to:  To points in Korea deemed nec
   WP date: 5 Apr 63
   Pd:      Approx 60 days
   Scty clnc: As indic
   Purpose: Stars & Stripes Actv
   Auth:    EUSA Cir 310-10
   Acct clas: NA
   Sp instr: Tvl by govt auto mil acft and ry dir.  Tvl perf under this
             O const dy contem by para 4250.3 JTR.  Govt rats and qtrs will
             be prov for pds of tvl and TDY dir by this O.
```

Special Order No. 72

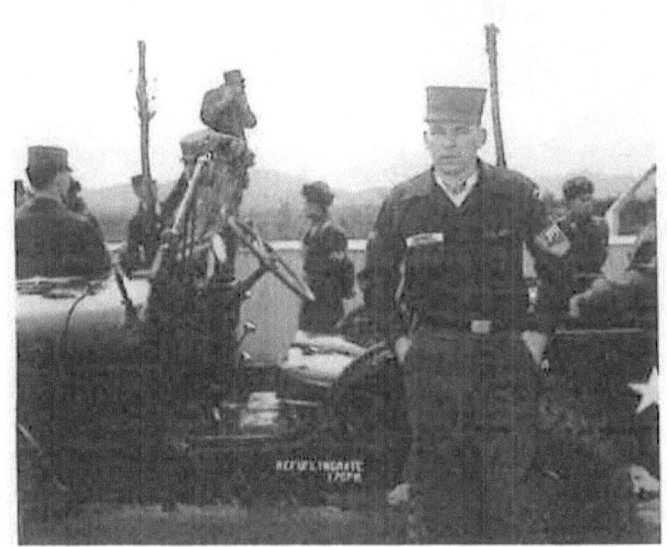

Panmunjom 1962. Standing beside my Jeep in the Joint Security Area (JSA). As the official United Nations Press Representative, I was one of the few non-security persons allowed to park inside the JSA. Directly behind me stand (to my right and left) two armed North Korean communist security guards. Note PRESS armband on my left arm.

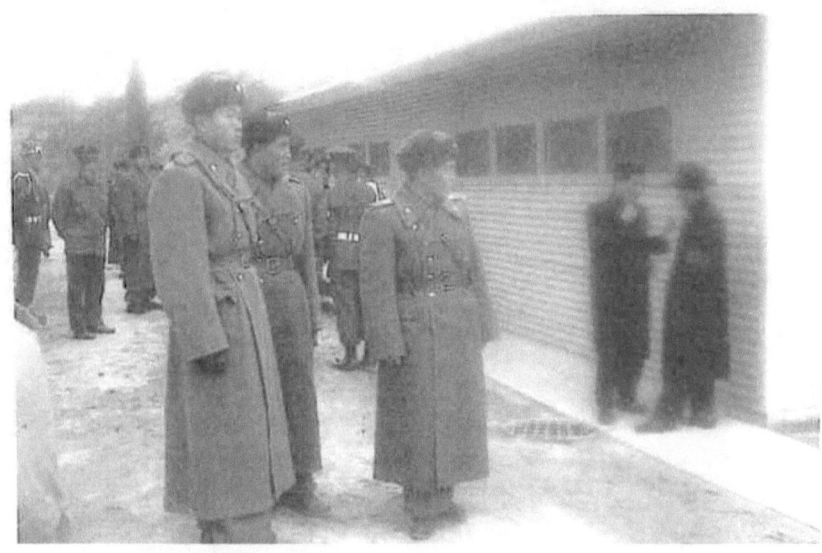

Panmunjom 1962. Inside the Joint Security Area (JSA). In the foreground stand three armed North Korean communist security guards. Note the ankle-length woolen coats. In the event of a firefight it would be nigh onto impossible for the communist security guards to run for cover.

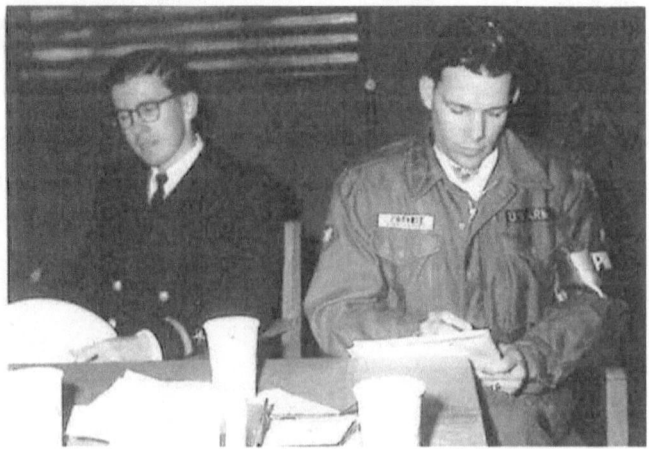

Panmunjom, Winter1962. Seated beside a U.S. Navy officer inside the Joint Security Area (JSA) Press Room, listening via a speaker attached to the wall inside, to the meeting taking place inside the Quonset hut next door.

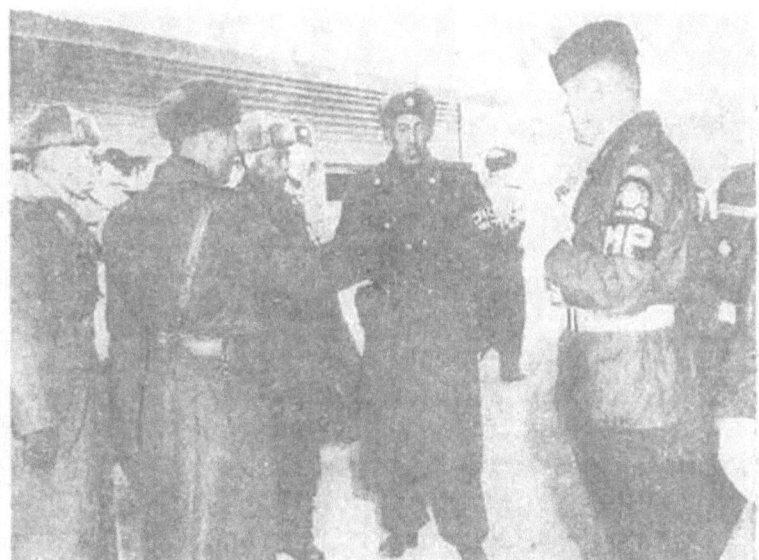

In an incident reflecting the tension at Panmunjom, Korea, scene of Military Armistice Commission meetings, U.S. Army Capt. Cecil N. Neely eyes communist guards who had gathered menacingly around an unidentified U.S. guard (far right). The communist in the center claimed the American guard bumped him. The Reds dispersed after Neely stepped in the way and other American guards gathered around. (USA Photo)

Panmunjom, Korea. Winter 1962. Confrontation between U.S. Army MPs and North Korean soldiers, while the meeting of the Military Armistice Commission is taking place in the large Quonset hut in the background. See caption of photo in *Stars & Stripes* article.

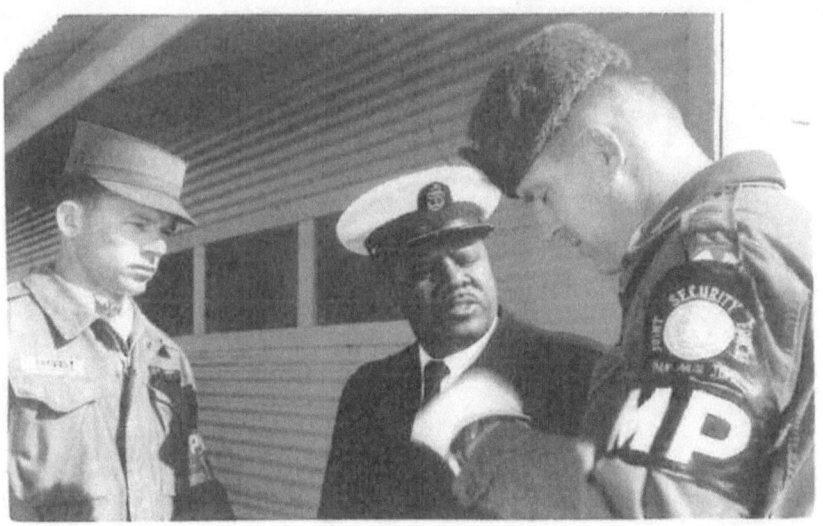

Panmunjom, summer of 1962. Following the altercation between the American and communist MPs, a U.S. Navy Chief Petty Officer and I listen as U.S. Army Captain Cecil N. Neely explains just how close we came to being caught up in a deadly shootout with 35 armed North Korean soldiers.

Chapter 9

◇◇◇◇

Return to Camp Page
(The Honest John Rocket Revisited)

When I joined the newspaper staff in early April 1962, one of the many situations about which Sergeant Kelsey cautioned me concerned the effect of the spring rains on the roads, ninety-five percent of which were of unpaved dirt, causing driving the large deuce-and-a-half troop transports to become a treacherous, downright tricky challenge. Jeeps fared little better.

And because of a dearth of funds available to pave them, roads often were carved into the sides of the steep Sorak mountains just waiting for the heavy rains to wash them away. It was accepted as a way of life in Korea.

I alone chose the stories I wanted to write. One of these had to do with proving to myself my suspicions that the Honest John Rocket was a *nuclear* and not a *conventional* weapon.

However this knowledge sought was strictly for my own edification. No way would I ever write a newspaper article about a nuclear weapon. Nor would I ever wish to do so.

In addition the trip would be a homecoming of sorts. I had spent a little more than two months with the guys in my unit prior to my *escape*, and knew them well enough to be welcomed back to Camp Page as a friend.

The only possible downside to my trip would be if I inadvertently ran into my nemesis, the colonel who commanded Camp Page and who would hate my guts forever for abandoning my duties as the post projectionist the moment I had earned my projectionist's "wings." He had taken my departure as a personal insult.

So I telephoned the major with whom I had established a friendship during the field exercises that had already been in progress upon my arrival at Camp Page back on January 3, 1962.

I explained to the major that I had been asked to do a story about Camp Page and the Honest John Rocket, except that we needed an actual photograph of the missile as it was being readied for launching.

The major assured me that this would not be a problem, and he told me when they had scheduled the upcoming field exercises.

With knowledge of the poor mountain roads made downright treacherous by the heavy spring rainfalls in mind, shortly after my arrival at the newspaper I wrote a story on the weather in Korea, with a focus on the intermittent heavy rainfall.

The U.S. Air Force weathermen had liked the story I wrote about them and were impressed by the way I had made a subject as dull as the weather into a halfway interesting newspaper article. As a result they encouraged me to telephone them for an up-to-date weather report anytime I would be taking a road trip.

Weather forecasting in Korea was the responsibility of U.S. Air Force's Detachment 18, First Weather Wing, headquartered in Seoul, where the forecasting was performed by Captain Paul R. Balcom and First Lieutenant Douglas D. Aho.

Four observation stations near Uijongbu in the DMZ recorded the weather information, which was in turn transmitted to Osan Air Base south of Seoul.

My plan had been to drive my Jeep from Seoul to Chunchon on Sunday, arriving at Camp Page by mid-afternoon, with my visit to the site of the simulated firings of the Honest John Rocket scheduled for the following morning. Assuming all went well weather-wise of course.

I telephoned my weathermen and gave them my itinerary for the following two days. The actual site of the planned rocket-simulated firing was about forty miles from Camp Page, up the rugged Sorak Mountain range. The convoy from Camp Page was scheduled to depart early, towing the rocket components behind several heavy troop transports.

The deployment and actual simulated firing of the Honest John Rocket was a team effort involving my old unit, the First Missile Battalion,

42ⁿᵈ Artillery, Fourth Missile Command, headquartered at Camp Page, and its sister unit from Camp Kaiser, Task Force Alpha (TFA).

On the way to the deployment site the rocket and warhead are transported aboard separate carriers. On site the rocket and warhead are mated and the rocket is then transferred from the *pull vehicle* to the launcher.

The weathermen informed me of an approaching weather front, but assured me this front, that had stalled off to the west over Seoul and Inchon, would not reach Chunchon until the day *after* the simulated rocket firing. This prediction was good enough for me, and I made preparations to leave early the following morning for Chunchon.

The weathermen's positive prediction however, seemed to hit a snag shortly before noon, and by mid-afternoon a light rain had begun to fall. But for the most part the rain let up throughout Sunday night.

I stayed at Camp Page that night. After breakfast the following morning the convoy of troop carriers departed Chunchon, pulling behind them the heavy components of the Honest John Rocket.

Bringing up the rear were two more heavy troop carriers, with me in my Jeep being the last vehicle in the convoy. A light rain was falling, and had been doing so throughout the night. What we did not know at the time, nor had we any warning, was that the light but steady rainfall had loosened the dirt that was the road that had been carved into the side of the mountain recently.

In all there were six heavy troop carriers in the convoy. The weight of each troop carrier had loosened the road bed that as I noted was nothing but dirt anyway.

And what is water in the form of rain, mixed with dirt? Why *mud* of course. Each of the heavy troop carriers in turn shifted the mud *away from* the side of the mountain and the road began to slowly slide down the mountain, to the extent that I feared the last two heavy troop transports might disappear down the steep mountain. What should I do? Do you mean before, or after, I had panicked?

The year was 1962. I had no way to contact the heavy troop carriers. And if the drivers attempted to turn around and reverse directions they too would slide down the steep mud bed. And the rainfall had increased in intensity.

I sounded the horn on my Jeep, that got the attention of the driver of the troop carrier about two hundred yards ahead of me. I began walking toward him while motioning him to come to me. We met on the road. I could tell by the look of concern on his face that the young driver wanted me to make the decisions.

"I'm going to drive back to Camp Page," I said. "I'll explain what's happened to the roadbed. Somebody will come with help. You all just wait here."

I turned my Jeep around and headed for Camp Page forty miles away. There was a light observation airplane based at a small hangar – little more than a shed really – inside Camp Page. I knew the pilot well because the hangar was located adjacent to the projectionist's building in one corner of the base.

Due to the light rainfall the pilot, a Warrant Officer, happened to be seated at his desk inside the small hangar that also served as his office. I explained the road situation to him and relayed my concerns about the weight of the troop transports coupled with the two large rocket components causing the roadbed to slowly slide down the mountain.

"Well grab your camera and let's go," he said. "This light rainfall won't bother the operation of my light observation plane because it is designed to fly in the rain."

Flying in from Chunchon heading east over the mountain range we first came to the last troop transport, that carried only troops. We continued flying toward the east until we came to two Jeeps, that carried the base commandant (my nemesis the colonel), and other officers who were to be part of the rocket simulation firing.

At this point the pilot told me that his best advice was to continue on to the demonstration site but have the troops alight from the troop transports when they encountered the treacherous sections.

"But what will happen when the exercise ends and the convoy must return to Camp Page?" I asked.

"This should not present a problem," said the pilot. "There is a return route. The distance is greater but the mountain is not as steep, so the convoy should make it safely back to Camp Page."

"What photos can I take to support your recommendation to continue heading east rather than turn around?" I asked.

Once again I, a lowly Specialist-4, found myself making decisions that were the province of a seasoned, high-ranking officer.

"We need a shot of a troop transport that shows the roadbed sliding off the side of the mountain. That should be all the proof we need."

"The next troop transport we see, turn toward the mountain, then bank around and I'll get a good shot that gets both the troop transport and the eroding roadbed in the picture," I said.

Shortly thereafter we saw our shot. The pilot headed toward the side of the mountain, then banked to our left. I looked out the small side window, took the shot, then took two more photos for good measure.

The pilot then flew low over the first two Jeeps in the convoy, the occupants being unaware of the problem of the roadbed sliding down the mountain. Not having his radio signal blocked by the mountains, the pilot established contact with the lead Jeep that carried – as my luck would have it – the commandant of Camp Page.

The pilot explained the roadbed problem and the fact that I had alerted him to the dangers of turning the convoy around.

"*Who* alerted you?" asked the colonel, who still apparently was holding a grudge against me.

"Provost," said the pilot. "He came up from Seoul to write a story about the rocket field exercise, and when he saw what was happening he drove back to Camp Page in his Jeep. We flew back here to warn you, and Provost took some photos to document everything."

"Well thank Provost for his quick thinking," said the colonel. "We'll contact the other vehicles in the convoy and take your advice about continuing on rather than turning around. I sure would like to see Provost's photos though."

At this point I quickly pressed my index finger to my lips in a silent plea that the pilot not mention the fact I was inside the airplane. I didn't want the colonel to feel as though he was obliged to speak to me. And truth be told I certainly did not wish to speak to him.

The pilot and I flew on to the site of the demonstration. He landed the light observation aircraft on a grassy field. Two hours later the convoy arrived and the Honest John Rocket team set up the simulated firing demonstration.

Mindful to stay out of the camp commandant's way, I snapped several photos of the technical team preparing the rocket for simulated firings.

During the course of these goings-on I did observe what I expected to see. Had the Honest John Rocket employed a conventional warhead, surely the technicians would have carried out an *actual* test firing. However no such firing ever took place, thus bolstering my theory that the Honest John Rocket carried a tactical nuclear warhead. At least on that occasion.

I did a short interview with the major whom I had befriended, and he divulged as much about the field exercise and the rocket as possible under the circumstances. Then I said goodbye to some friends I had soldiered with on my initial two-month tour at Camp Page back in January 1962. Then the pilot and I climbed into his plane and flew back to Chunchon. I thanked the pilot for his assistance and three hours later I reached the Seoul city limits. All in all my assignment to Camp Page had been successful.

One of the few rules set down by Colonel Creel when I joined the newspaper staff in early April 1962 was that I had to alert him whenever I was going to write a story that mentioned specific weapons of any kind. I wrote the story my way. Then I dropped a typed copy by the colonel's office.

As a result sometimes the stories would appear in the newspaper except that half or more had been deleted. Therefore I pushed the technical and weapons aspect of the story, wondering whether I would ever see any of it in print.

This time however I got lucky. Well, sort of anyway. The censors had deleted more than half the printed story and several of the photos that showed very close-up views of the rocket itself.

However I was pleased with the two photos that were included with the final abbreviated article. One photo showed the warhead of the rocket being "married" to the body of the rocket. But the best shot was the aerial photo showing the large troop carrier beginning its slide down the muddy, precarious Sorok Mountain road.

On my drive from Chunchon to Seoul after leaving the pilot, I reasoned that although I had alerted the pilot to the impending disaster, it was the pilot who had given the officers of Camp Page advice on the best way to reach their destination without damage to the Honest John Rocket components and the heavy troop carriers.

Truth be told my heart was in my throat praying that the driver of the troop transport in the *Stars & Stripes* photo would not slide to his death as he negotiated that sharp bend on the muddy road that day.

The Versatile Honest John Rocket

The MGR-1 Honest John Rocket was the first *nuclear-capable* surface-to-surface missile in the United States military arsenal. The rocket was first tested on June 29, 1951, with the first production rounds being delivered in January 1953.

The Honest John was a large, fin-stabilized *unguided* artillery rocket that weighed 5,820 pounds in its M-31 nuclear-armed version. It was mounted on the back of a truck, aimed the same way as a cannon, then fired up an elevated ramp. Sounded almost archaic; however it was considered state-of-the-art at the time.

With a 20 kiloton *nuclear* warhead its range was 15.4 miles, and it was also capable of carrying a 1500 pound *conventional* warhead. The major problem encountered in its development was increased scatter-on-target because of it being an *unguided* missile. Improvements over the years increased its maximum range to greater than 30 miles.

Although the Honest John was unguided and was the first U.S. nuclear ballistic missile, it had a longer life than all other U.S. ballistic missiles except Minuteman. The total number produced was more than 7,000.

In 1973 the system was replaced with the MGM-52 Lance missile. However it was deployed with National Guard units in the United States until 1982 and with NATO units in Europe until 1985. Standing within fifty yards of the Honest John in its ready-to-fire position, the best word used to describe the weapon would be "menacing."

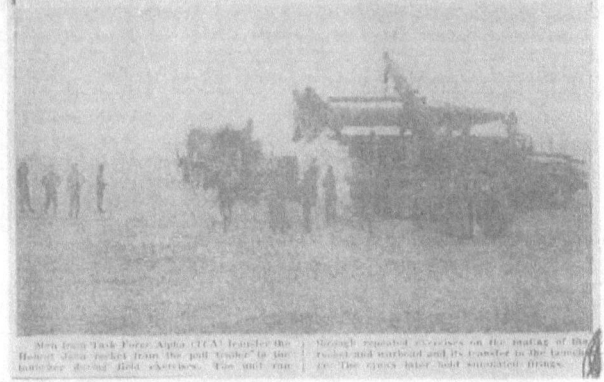

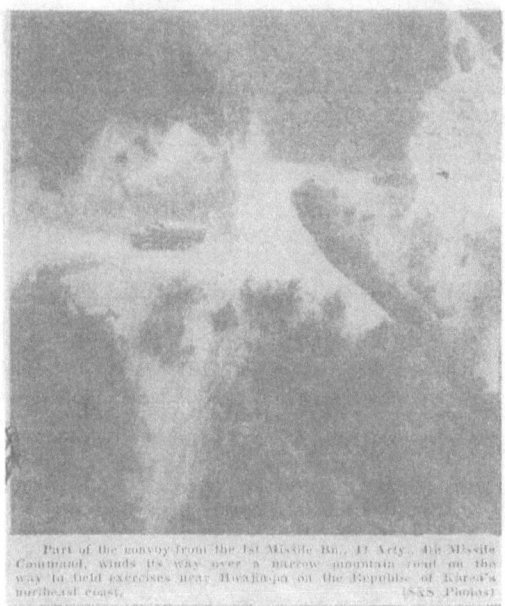

Summer of 1962. Note: There are two photos here.

  I. Summer 1962. (Use the caption from the Stars & Stripes that shows the missile being assembled.)

  II. Summer of 1962 (Use the caption from the Stars & Stripes that shows the aerial view of the side of the mountain.)

Chapter 10

◇◇◇◇◇

The Drowned Communist Spy Inside The Japanese Midget Submarine

The last two weeks in November 1962 were wet and cold (i.e., miserable) across the Korean peninsula. I had used my time wisely, researching and writing some interesting stories on a variety of subjects and happenings of both a civilian and military nature. And loving every minute of it.

Along the way I had increased the number of freelance stories I was selling to stateside newspapers, keeping a notebook showing the name of the stateside newspaper, title of the article, date payment received and the amount received for the article.

In keeping with the advice I had received from the other reporters, I simply mailed the article, including the related photographs, along with a letter and a copy of the article that I had written for the *Stars & Stripes*, to the editor of the stateside hometown newspaper.

I never asked for payments of any amount. Newspapers have a set "scale" for freelance work. The checks I received for my stories generally were for $50, sometimes a little more but never less. The freelance business was good.

As discussed earlier, because I was the only reporter who possessed a Top Secret Security Clearance, from time to time I would receive instructions from Col. George Creel, head of the U.S. Eighth Army Information Office, to contact a certain high-ranking officer concerning a story, sensitive in nature, that the officer requested that I write.

As usual I was to investigate and write the story but instead of turning it in to my Bureau Chief Sergeant Kelsey, I was to deliver the only copy to Col. Creel after the requesting officer reviewed the story for factual accuracy.

In such cases of course, Col. Creel was acting in his capacity as censor for the army. More often than not however, if there were questions concerning the sensitivity of the subject matter the colonel would choose to kick the story up to G-2 at the Pentagon in Washington, D.C., deftly taking himself out of the loop.

In the course of my fifteen months at the *Stars & Stripes*, only one of the seven such stories I wrote ever made it to the pages of the newspaper.

If only the public knew what it was missing!

Anyway during the second week in November 1962 heavy rainfall commenced, causing the normally fast-moving river along the DMZ, over which spanned the notorious *Bridge of No Return*, to greatly increase its already treacherous flow. The DMZ troops called the raging river the *Mean Mother*.

A week after the rains abated I received a call from Col. Creel. I was to travel that very day to the headquarters of the U.S. First Cavalry Division, known among soldiers in South Korea as the "First Cav," and check in with a certain named colonel.

At the time of this call I happened to be at my desk proofreading an article I was preparing to submit to Sergeant Kelsey. I told Kelsey where I was going, grabbed my poncho in case it rained, jammed my wrapped .38 Special beneath the driver's seat of my trusty Jeep and two hours later was checking in at the headquarters of the First Cavalry Division. The colonel had been expecting me. He quickly introduced himself.

"How can I help you colonel?" I said.

Blinking in mild surprise the colonel asked the same question I had heard a half-dozen times.

"And they sent you, son?" As though there had been some mistake in communication.

"Let's drive over to that large tent that has been set up over yonder," he said pointing out the window in the direction of "yonder.

Minutes later we were walking into the tent and into a scene that appeared surreal, almost unworldly, definitely a shock to the senses. Several senior officers were bending over a long table inspecting the bloated and discolored body of a Korean male who appeared to have been wearing clothes six sizes too small.

"Looks like he drowned several days ago, when the river overflowed its banks and flipped the submarine over on its side," explained a major.

"Yes," added another major. "When we first lifted the sub out of the river it was filled with water."

"What kind of submarine is this," I asked. "I've never seen a sub as small as this." (Or any sub for that matter.)

As I asked the question one of the officers reached for a thick book lying on the table.

"We've never seen one of these on this river before," he said. "They're called Japanese *midget* subs. Usually each sub will hold one or two persons, together with the appropriate armament and batteries and motor for propulsion."

"We have a book here that describes some of these submarines," said the officer opening the book to a marked page. We can show it to you because of your Top Secret Clearance. You do have such clearance, don't you soldier?" The half-dozen officers standing around the body of the North Korean laughed good-naturedly.

"I can see there are several empty compartments here," I said, squatting and peering into the sub's conning tower. "What was in these compartments?"

"Apparently there was room for a second man. This would account for one large empty compartment. And because this was a spy mission designed to infiltrate South Korea, he had no need for the two large torpedoes, the scuttling charge or most of the ballast."

"Then it would appear that he intended to make a return trip," I said. "Like he was delivering something valuable that he was ensuring would not fall into our hands."

"I believe you are correct," said the major, walking over to another table and pointing first at a stack of papers, then at two stacks of currency, one of hundred dollar bills and another in South Korean *won*.

"The American money is $20,000 in hundreds and the second is $20,000 in *won*," he said.

"Then the dead Korean is simply a courier, don't you reckon?" I asked.

"We agree with you," said the major. "We'll deliver the stack of papers to the 502 Military Intelligence Battalion in Seoul. Between those intel guys and the two CIA agents on the compound they'll figure out what it's all about."

"Could you answer a question for me?" I asked without thinking.

"That's why you're here, so just ask away," he said.

"Have you ever seen one of these midget subs before?"

"Personally none of us has ever seen one of them," he answered. "We have been told however that two years ago, again during a heavy rain, a North Korean agent drowned on this same river."

"Can I get inside the sub to take some photos?" I asked expectantly.

"The sub is 78 feet long and 10 feet in height. But we had trouble pulling the bloated body out, and had to spray against disease. So it's best if you could just stick your camera inside and snap your photos. Is this all right with you?"

"This will not be a problem," I said.

So I took two rolls of film with my 35mm Nikon and flash, while remarking (under my breath, of course) that not one line of type or a single photograph would ever see the inside of the *Stars & Stripes*. Absolutely not.

When I began my career at the newspaper, Col. Creel encouraged me to state my opinion on the story before submitting it to him. "If the higher-ups trust you enough to give you a Top Secret Clearance, you should be able to analyze the facts and offer an intelligent opinion." he said.

After I had taken the photos I copied some of the nomenclature of the sub into my small pocket notebook I always carried with me.

The sub was a *Type A Ko-hyoteki-class* submarine. A total of 101 had been manufactured by the Japanese prior to the attack on Pearl Harbor on December 7, 1941. Several of the subs had been used in that surprise attack. Apparently the North Koreans seized some of the subs at the end of World War II in August 1945.

The subs were 78' 5" in length and 9' 10" high at the conning tower. Their speeds were 26 MPH surfaced and 22 MPH submerged, about the speed of the average bicyclist. They had been depth-tested at 98 feet. Each was armed with two 17.7-inch-long torpedoes muzzle-loaded into tubes, and one 300-pound scuttling charge.

I had driven through a light rain from Seoul to First Cav headquarters earlier that morning for the meeting with the colonel, three majors and a captain.

By 1:00 p.m. I had finished gathering material and taking photographs for my (never-to be-published) article, and the light rain had petered out to no rain.

I informed the colonel that I could make it back to Seoul before nightfall, and he suggested we all walk over to the officers' mess hall for lunch, then I could be on my way. A few more questions would round out my article.

"You told me the North Korean likely drowned after the submarine tipped over on its side?" I asked.

"Yes," said a major. "One of the M.P.s on patrol up at *The Bridge of No Return* observed a long metal object sticking up out of the river following the heavy rainfall. Let's drive over to the river and I'll show you where we found the submarine."

Ten minutes later the officers and I stood on the banks of the still raging river. The view was a shock to my senses. Raging mountain rivers do not flow in straight lines, and I knew at first glance that there was no way the sub could keep from capsizing in such a strong current. Only a fool would believe otherwise.

In addition it would be a one-way trip. A week after the rainfall ceased the current was still so swift that it would have been impossible for the Japanese minisub to travel *upstream*. It had been a suicide mission from the outset.

There is no way to explain the inexplicable using the principles of logic. At this moment I was dying to ask one of my friends at the 502 the couple of dozen questions I had concerning the incident. But then I recalled Jon Powell's admonition about "talking shop" concerning the workings of the 502.

Thus for the moment at least, I was stymied in my quest for learning the reason the communists would attempt such a foolhardy mission. Perhaps I would find out later.

The scene I viewed upon entering the large hospital tent has been with me forever. The bloated body of the communist spy. The garish death mask with the protruding eyes. The body splotched in various shades of brown, blue and black. The stretched skin of the torso, reminding me of the expression, "Jumping out of his skin from fright."

All of these descriptions together encompass a futuristic, almost unworldly scene, straight out of a Boris Karloff horror movie.

If I were to state the one quality that has made me a success in almost any endeavor in life, it would be the fact that I was – and still am – always thinking. My transmission of life is definitely missing a *Neutral* gear.

Therefore by the time I had completed the two-hour return trip from First Cav headquarters to the *Stars & Stripes* Press Room and living quarters, I had already written, proofread and rewritten one of my favorite stories that I knew never would see the pages of the *Stars & Stripes*.

That night I typed my story and the following morning carried the article and film into the Eighth U.S. Army Headquarters to Col. Creel.

"Okay Provost," said the colonel after he had read my story. "I like it, and I'm looking forward to seeing the photos. I'll let you know whether we get past the censors."

I left Col. Creel's office with little hope. The drowned communist spy had to be high on the *military-sensitive scale*. All I could do was to wait and see.

Three days later I received a telephone call from Col. Creel.

"Provost, your photos were fascinating. You did a good job with the story also. But despite this, the army censors decided the story was a *No Go*."

"Did they offer a reason?" I asked.

"The North Korean mission failed of course. But printing the story will alert them to this fact. So by not writing the story the communists will be kept in the dark as to whether the mission was successful or not."

I suppose I could live with this explanation. However I still wish they had printed my story.

The Bridge of No Return

We lowly mortals are saddled with oodles of phobias. We don't defeat them. It's just that we are so frightened of them, we hope that by not speaking of them out loud they will disappear. Foolish mortals, we.

The First Cavalry Division's first line of defense required to blunt an invasion across the DMZ from North Korea is actually not a military fortification but a wide, mean, raging river just about kissing the DMZ, not far from the small town of Uijongbu, South Korea. See included photo. It's the same river in which the pilot of the Japanese mini sub drowned. Foolish communists, they.

Now the demolitions company of the First Cav could blow the bridge anytime it received an order. However, the bridge and the river are both situated on the South Korean part of land, and some units of the First Cav are stationed north of the river. What makes these troops uneasy is that in the event the North Koreans launch an attack at this point and dynamite the long bridge, these units would be trapped north of the river. So here's the problem, and it's a real one.

Many years ago there were two bridges, one for the vehicular traffic and the other for train traffic. However, the vehicular bridge was destroyed, leaving a narrow, one-way-only bridge. Large wooden planks now make up the bed, and because it was intended to carry train traffic only, the plank roadbed has enough room for but one vehicle at a time to travel the long length of the bridge. The Americans dubbed the span *The Bridge of No Return* because in the event of war likely only a portion of the U.S. troops would be able to escape to safety across the narrow bridge.

The One-star's Big Mistake

Except in rare instances, as the *Stars & Stripes* only feature writer I had my choice as to the stories I wanted to cover. When I came aboard I asked Jon Powell and Bureau Chief Sergeant Kelsey what they would like to see me write.

"Provost, if you write about what interests you, you'll be in the ball park ninety percent of the time," said Kelsey.

"Come to think of it," said Powell, "I don't believe anyone has covered one of the First Cav's Rifle and Pistol Competitions this year. You'd probably like to spend a few hours up along the DMZ Provost, interviewing some of the best marksmen in the U.S. Army."

Sounded like a good idea to me, so I telephoned First Cavalry Division Headquarters and was patched through to a captain who appeared to be knowledgeable about the subject matter. He gave me the particulars concerning the upcoming rifle matches and I made plans to attend.

Now the nice captain was not exactly dealing with a novice. My first DD Form 214 included a statement that I had been awarded a *Marksman's Badge* in similar competition.

Each of the four major branches of the military has its own standard as to what qualifies for a Marksman's Badge and a Sharpshooter's Badge. In the early 1960s to be awarded a Marksman's Badge the shooter had to hit 26 out of 30 pop-up targets at a specified distance. So I knew my way around firearms.

The competition was open to the best shooters who had defeated others to reach the finals. I took a lot of photos and met some of the best shots in the First Cavalry Division.

The competition ended at 4:00 p.m., and several hundred soldiers watched the commanding general as he prepared to present the awards. I was seated on the first row of bleachers, holding one of my 35mm Nikons at the ready, with my second fully-loaded camera hanging by a leather strap around my neck.

"Stand up, soldier!" barked the stern-faced general, who seemed to be speaking to someone in my general vicinity.

The general could not have been addressing me, I assumed, because I was merely a newspaper reporter. So I remained seated.

"I mean *you*, soldier, the one with the camera strap around your neck. Stand up."

"Yes, sir," I said hesitantly, debating as to whether I should try to explain myself. I stood, staring straight ahead. I decided to keep my mouth shut.

"What's your name, soldier?" The voice just as demanding, just as caustic.

"Specialist Fourth Class Al Provost," sir.

"You're out of uniform, Provost," the general said. "Don't you ever show up here again out of uniform. Now sit down."

"Yes, sir," I said. I sat. Very quietly.

It's hardly worth mentioning at this point, but I cannot fault the embarrassed captain for not coming to my defense, for to do so would have in turn embarrassed the Brigadier General. And this would never do.

The captain walked me to my Jeep for my return south to Seoul.

"Well I would understand it if you didn't print any of the photos," he said. "I'm sorry this happened to you."

"I suppose I'll print the photos, sir. My Bureau Chief knows this is where I was coming, and what happened was not the fault of any of the soldiers. However as long as the general is the commanding officer here, I'll never return."

"Well hopefully you and I will meet again," he said. "The general is scheduled to rotate stateside in four months. I'll give you a call at the newspaper office in Seoul when he leaves."

I was happy to receive a call from the captain four months later. The U.S. Army's First Calvary Division defended a large swath of real estate immediately south of the DMZ. A lot of good stories in that large area of land. And the camera hanging from the leather strap around my neck was a dead giveaway.

The Case of the Envious Captain

When I arrived at the *Stars & Stripes* office in early April 1962 as the new feature writer, our nine-man unit was *commanded* – if one could call it that – by a Second Lieutenant, the lowest-ranking officer who, lo and behold, possessed only a *Secret* Security Clearance.

Aside from showing his displeasure at the fact that I possessed a security clearance higher than that of his own, for the most part the young lieutenant stayed out of my way – and I his. One might call our relationship *an impasse*.

One morning in late August 1962 I was seated at my desk in the Press Room typing my latest (no doubt Pulitzer Prize-winning) gem when I looked up to see a U.S. Army captain enter the front door.

Sergeant Kelsey and a few of the other reporters were in the Press Room at the time, and we all stood and saluted the captain smartly. He returned our salute, said "At ease. As you were," and I returned to my typing.

The captain turned to Sergeant Kelsey.

Author's note: So as to avoid embarrassing anyone, the only time I will use a person's real name is if he or she is one of the good guys. This seems appropriate to me. Thus I will use a fictitious name for the captain and will refer to him as *Captain Morgan*. He was at this time addressing our Bureau Chief Warren Kelsey. His real name, thus one of the good guys.

"Sergeant Kelsey," began Captain Morgan, quickly reading the name tag on Kelsey's shirt. "I'm Captain Morgan. I just yesterday took over as the C.O. (Commanding Officer) of the *Stars & Stripes* from the lieutenant."

"I'm very pleased to meet you Captain Morgan," said the always polite and ever respectful Bureau Chief from Tennessee. The men shook hands cordially.

"Sergeant, if this were a larger unit I couldn't do this, but because there seems to be only eight or nine of us, I'd like to meet with each of you for a few minutes in private, sort of a *meet-and-greet* like we used to have at the beginning of our classes in law school."

Immediately I picked up on the "law school" reference. The captain must have been at least in his mid-thirties, and if he had graduated law school and passed the Bar examination, what was he doing in Korea "commanding" eight enlisted men?

Thus the only explanation was that he had graduated law school but failed to pass the Bar examination. At least three times.

In 1962 a law school graduate was permitted to take the Bar exam only three times. If he or she still failed it after three attempts, he or she was precluded from sitting for it again. This was what had happened to the captain.

However this was no concern of mine, and I actually sympathized with him. I knew however that when the next copies of the TDY (Temporary Duty) orders, that came out from Eighth U.S. Army headquarters once every 60 days, arrived at the *Stars & Stripes* compound, the captain would see that I was the only reporter who possessed a Top Secret Security Clearance. And like several officers before him, this slighted captain surely would see that my security clearance ranked above that of his own.

Egads! This Top Secret Security Clearance was fast becoming a liability, my own personal albatross.

Truer words, and all that follows. I was the last of the eight men interviewed, and as soon as I entered Captain Morgan's office I noticed a copy of our TDY orders resting on the desk before him.

"I'm curious, Provost. Sergeant Kelsey tells me you are the newspaper's only feature writer. How does this differ from just a reporter?"

"As the feature writer I am assigned my own Jeep. I travel throughout South Korea, writing about what interests me. I do not work under a fixed schedule."

"Who made you the feature writer? Why, you're one of the youngest reporters."

"Col. Creel, head of the Eighth Army Information Office, gave me the job of feature writer when I came here from the Fourth Missile Command in Chunchon back in April of this year."

"So you say you write what you want to write about?"

"Yes, sir, but sometimes Col. Creel sends me on special assignments."

"Such as?" he asked quizzically.

"That would be classified, sir." A long pause ensued, as though he was not certain I had said what he thought I had actually said. He continued.

"What else do you write about?"

"I must attend every meeting of the Military Armistice Commission, held in the Joint Security Area of the DMZ."

"How often are these meetings held?"

"They average at least one per month, sometimes twice. Every time the thin-skinned Chinese or North Koreans get their feelings hurt, they demand a meeting. But I must cover every meeting regardless of whether I think it has merit."

"Why is this?"

"Because Col. Creel and Sergeant Kelsey have found my writing to be clear, concise and factually correct. In other words they trust me."

But the captain could not get his mind off the fact that some stories I was asked to write were classified. So he pressed the point.

"What are some subjects that would be classified?"

"Anything that involves weapons, their use and capabilities, in particular weapons systems being tested. If a commander wishes us to give the weapon some publicity, Col. Creel will ask me to write the story, but I'm to return the typewritten story to Col. Creel to have the censors review it before it appears in the newspaper."

"You must be one of the youngest reporters on the newspaper," he said. "How old are you?"

"I'm 22 years old, sir, and I am indeed the youngest reporter."

"But how did you come to have a Top Secret Security Clearance?"

"I received a Top Secret Security Clearance two weeks after I graduated from college. I enlisted in the U.S. Army two weeks later, on June 30, 1961."

"What did you major in in undergraduate school?"

"Physics and mathematics, a double major, with a Concentration in Atomic Physics."

"And where have you been stationed since you joined the army?"

"Basic Infantry Training at Ft. Jackson, South Carolina. Advanced Artillery Training at Ft. Sill, Oklahoma. U.S. Fourth Missile Command, Chunchon, Korea."

"So you went through all this technical training on weapons systems, and then they send you to be a feature writer for a newspaper? Why would the army do this?"

"Sir the *reason* I received a Top Secret Security Clearance when I was but two weeks out of college is itself a Top Secret matter, and I would be in violation of my clearance if I discussed the subject further. Suffice it to say that when I joined the army I agreed to go where the army ordered me to go. I suggest if you desire more information you should contact Col. Creel."

I had tried my best not to insult the captain. However the fact was that I, a lowly Specialist-4, possessed a Top Secret Security Clearance whereas he, a captain, had been granted but a Secret Security Clearance. We were not destined to become bosom buddies.

With Captain Morgan I had tried my best to avoid conflict, to not ruffle his feathers, to "get along" so to speak.

However he couldn't seem to be able to come to grips with the situation. I sensed trouble a-brewing, and believed he would seek to do me harm if events allowed him an opening.

Because of my feelings, as soon as I found the time I telephoned Col. Creel and explained the conversation I had with the captain. The colonel told me to keep him informed, and I hoped things would improve.

They didn't.

In order to avoid trouble I attempted the same tact I had used with the previous commander, the Second Lieutenant – I kept out of his way.

This did not take much effort on my part. Just like the departed Second Lieutenant, Captain Morgan did not live inside the *Stars & Stripes* two-story building that, as previously noted, was a converted Korean all-brick warehouse. Rather every day during the work week, at around 3:00 p.m. he would drive to his officers' quarters on Eighth U.S. Army headquarters at Yongsan, where he billeted.

The Vindictive Captain Sees an Opening

The vaunted U.S. First Cavalry Division (The "First Cav") was strung out along the lower (southernmost) section of the Demilitarized Zone (DMZ). The First Cav's mission was to blunt any invasion by the North Korean Army.

As I could readily attest based on the number of articles that appeared under my byline in the *Stars & Stripes* during the period April 1962-July 1963, the officers and enlisted men of the First Cav took their mission seriously. They trained and trained and trained, after which they trained some more.

And because they covered such a large area, the M.P.s would throw up a roadblock at the blink of an eye, stopping cold all vehicular traffic until I.D.s of all drivers (and passengers) were checked. And within three or four weeks of my arrival at the *Stars & Stripes* compound in Seoul, the M.P.s manning these checkpoints recognized me and my Jeep and simply waved me through.

I owe my success in life to the fact that I have always been thinking. At no time do I allow my mind's transmission to slip into neutral. I never ever forget anything, trust me.

Except…

Except for the morning I was in a hurry to get to a unit in the First Cav located right along the DMZ, and forgot my billfold resting on my nightstand at the newspaper office. And what was contained in this billfold? Why, nothing of great importance I suppose.

Except for my military driver's license. And except for my United Nations Command laminated Press Pass, that under normal conditions cautioned anyone reading the card not to interfere with me in the furtherance of my duties. Both cards contained my photograph.

Oblivious to my error, I was simply waved through two north bound traffic stops, and three hours later, having written my story and taken my photographs I was once again heading south.

Except that there were two M.P.s manning the roadblock, not the same ones who had been there on my way north early that morning. Not to worry though because I recognized both of them. Therefore they surely knew me. Didn't work out that way though.

"Okay Provost," said one M.P. "Let me see your driver's license. It'll only take a minute."

It took me two seconds tops to determine I did not have my billfold and thus had neither my driver's license nor my press pass card. Damn!

"How stupid of me," I said – and meant it. "In my hurry to get up here to write my story I just left it on my nightstand. I'm sorry. How can I make it right?"

"It shouldn't be a problem Provost," he responded. "Just sit here and I'll telephone your unit commander. He'll okay us giving you a temporary driver's license and you can be on your way."

Ever have one of those little "situations" in life that start out bad and end up worse? This was one of those situations.

Well anyway I went inside the M.P. station to wait while the M.P. telephoned the newspaper office and spoke with Captain Morgan. After what I thought was an inordinately long period of time for such a routine, simple request, the M.P. emerged from the rear office. He was not smiling.

"My god what a hardass," he began. "What's the captain got against you, Provost?"

I briefly explained the story of the Top Secret Clearance. "And he's got a problem with a lowly Spec-4 having a Top Secret Clearance when he, a hotshot captain, doesn't have one. So what do I have to do to get on my way to Seoul?"

"The son of a bitch won't authorize us to give you a temporary driver's license. He says you'll have to take the army bus to Seoul, pick up your driver's license, then take the bus back up here, show us your driver's license, pick up your Jeep and drive on back to Seoul. He said he was doing this to teach you a lesson. What a miserable bastard."

It was getting on late in the day. I left my Jeep in the parking lot, waited longer than an hour to catch the last bus of the day heading to Seoul and arrived at the *Stars & Stripes* office after sundown.

The following morning I caught the 10:00 a.m. bus from Seoul to the First Cav, showed my driver's license to the M.P.s, then arrived back in Seoul at 4:00 p.m. A wasted day.

I was greeted at the door of the Press Room by Sergeant Kelsey. The captain had already left for the day.

"I've already notified Col. Creel of what happened," said Kelsey. "He told me to let you know that he's going to take care of the problem."

And it took but a few weeks for Col. Creel to act. Captain Morgan usually had breakfast at the Yongsan compound in Seoul, then drove his Jeep to the newspaper office south of the Han River in the Yungdung po district of Seoul.

Not having any pressing duties waiting for him he rarely ever arrived at the office before 10:00 a.m. and by then I was already on the road doing my thing.

Then one day the other reporters, Sergeant Kelsey and I got dressed and walked around the corner to have breakfast at the 502 mess hall. After ordering from the young Korean waitress and each getting a mug of coffee, Sergeant Kelsey rose to speak. His ear-to-ear grin really said it all.

"You guys know what happened between the captain and Provost," he began. "And you also know I reported the incident to Col. Creel." There were nods of agreement all around.

"Did the colonel ever take any action?" asked one of the reporters. "Provost has been hiding out from the captain ever since then." The other reporters laughed because that was exactly what I had been doing. The less I saw of the vindictive captain, the better.

"Well anyway, don't expect to ever see the captain again. He left yesterday, having been reassigned to an infantry company somewhere close to the DMZ," responded Kelsey. "Col. Creel said to carry on and he would have a new unit commander within a week or two. So Provost, you can come out of hiding now. We'll likely never hear from your arrogant captain again."

But I did. Like a bloomin' bad penny he was.

During the hard winter months of December, January and February in Korea, the days are bitterly cold, with ice and snow for days on end. We might as well have been living in Buffalo, New York. I even thought of retiring my newspaper byline until April 1, 1963.

I recall it was an icy day in late December 1962. We all were seated at our desks inside the press room, already having decided we would not dare venture out in all that ice and snow. Possibly the following day. But probably not.

The telephone rang. Sergeant Kelsey lifted the receiver and held it to his ear.

"*Stars & Stripes*. Sergeant Kelsey here."

Kelsey listened intently for a few moments. Then he spoke, while at the same time fixing his gaze on me from across the room. His look was that of a curious newborn longhaired Persian.

"It's for you Provost," he said, extending the receiver to me.

"Who is it?" I asked in a low voice.

"You'll never guess," replied the bureau chief, holding his hand over the receiver.

The ensuring brief conversation went something like this:

Spec-4 Provost: Provost here. How can I help you?

Captain Morgan: Provost, this is Captain Morgan. How are you getting along with all this cold weather?

Spec-4 Provost: Trying my best to stay inside, sir. How are things with you, and by the way where are you now?

(As though I really cared.)

He gave me the name of the infantry unit he commanded. It was about as far north as you could go and still be in South Korea.

Spec4-Provost: My god, Captain Morgan, you must be freezing.

Captain Morgan: I am. I'm calling to ask a favor of you Provost.

Spec-4 Provost: Anything for you, Captain Morgan. Just ask away.

Captain Morgan: When you write a story for the *Stars & Stripes*, are you still writing the same story for the hometown newspaper?

Spec-4 Provost: Yes sir, I am. We call those "vanity pieces." Would you like for me to write a vanity piece for you, using your unit as the backdrop for the story?

Captain Morgan: I certainly would, Provost. When could you drive up to write the story? The sooner the better.

Spec-4 Provost: Well as you can tell with all the ice covering the roads, I'll have to wait for the weather to clear. Why don't you just wait for me to telephone you. Don't worry sir, I'll make you look good.

Captain Morgan: Okay Provost, I'll wait for your call. Don't wait too long.

When I turned to give the receiver to Kelsey, I noticed that Kelsey and the other reporters had been listening to my part of my conversation with the arrogant captain. The expressions on their faces matched that of my own.

"Well Provost, are you going to write the vanity piece and make the bastard look good?" asked one of the reporters.

"You know he's looking for a way out of that icebox called the DMZ, don't you?" asked another.

"After treating you the way he did?" asked a third. "He's got more nerve than the law allows."

A few weeks later, with the swirling north winds still colder'n a witch's tit, I telephoned Captain Morgan. The captain never had been big on preambles, especially when he wanted something.

"Well Provost, it's about time," were the first words out of his mouth. "When can you be here?" The attitude in his tone could only be characterized as "short." I pressed on.

"The reason I'm calling, Captain Morgan, is to let you know that all this ice and snow has really put us behind on the stories we have to write," I said with all the false sincerity I could muster. "All I can say is that I'll get to your story as soon as possible. And by the way sir, how has the weather been up along the DMZ lately?"

As dense as he was, he may not have picked up on that last nuance. Or perhaps he had, because I never heard from him again. Which was just fine with me.

Captain Morgan, the Proverbial Bad Penny True, I never heard *from* the pompous captain again. However I did hear *of* him. The pundits are correct after all; it really is a small world.

On November 4, 1965 I received an Honorable Discharge from the U.S. Army. In May 1972 I graduated from the University of Houston with a doctorate in Optometry (O.D.) and began practicing Optometry in Ft. Lauderdale, Florida.

In the fall of 1977 I began studying Law at Nova Southeastern University College of Law. In 1980 I graduated with a Doctorate of Laws (J.D.) degree. I took and passed the Bar in Georgia and Florida in 1980, and opened a law office in Ft. Lauderdale. All went well.

The Florida Bar publishes a newspaper every other week, filled with news relating to the practice of Law in Florida. Fast-forward to the year 1986, six years after I started my law practice.

I was sitting at my desk one morning when my secretary plopped the latest issue of the legal newspaper down on the corner of my desk. Not having anything to occupy my time at the moment, I picked up the newspaper and began perusing the articles.

Suddenly I experienced a not so mild shock to my senses. I blinked rapidly several times in an attempt to clear the image of someone I had last seen 24 years earlier, in 1962. Literally a ghost from my past – Captain Morgan.

The article printed beneath his photo related that Mr. Morgan, an associate in a Miami law firm, had been named to one of the Florida Bar's standing committees. But why was the captain – now a civilian – able to practice law when he had failed three times to pass the Florida Bar examination?

So I consulted the Florida Case Law and found the answer to my question. According to what Captain Morgan told me in 1962, the rule of the Florida Bar provided that if a lawyer could not pass the Bar exam in three tries, he likely would never become a lawyer.

However sometime during those 24 years, from 1962 to 1986, the rule had been changed, and in 1986 a lawyer could take the Bar exam for as many times as it took for him to pass it. So the captain had finally lucked out and passed the Bar. Silently I wished the captain well. Arrogance is a character flaw, not a sin.

Chapter 11

◇◇◇◇◇

The Offer I Couldn't Refuse

Within two months of my arrival at the *Stars & Stripes* two things of note had been added to my repertoire of experiences relating to Korea and its people, both having to do with my response to tiny but quite real phobias, as follows:

When I arrived at the newspaper on April 10, 1962 as the feature writer, Sergeant Kelsey offered me the services of Kim Ki Sam as both my photographer and interpreter.

Failing to see the challenge in this arrangement, I told Kelsey I would go it alone. The bureau chief's only admonition as I walked out the door on my very first assignment was, "Now don't you get lost, Provost."

My decision to memorize the map of Korea was mandated by this comment from our illustrious bureau chief, and my thoughts when I read the Legend of the only map Kelsey had given me, that stated I was holding in my (suddenly) sweaty palms a 1946 Japanese road map of Korea! My god, I thought, this blinkin' map was 16 years old (1946-1962) and had been surveyed by a country that had come out on the short end of the bloodiest war in recorded history!

The only way to ensure I never would make a wrong turn and stumble into communist North Korea would be to locate an accurate map of South Korea and memorize it. Which I did, as soon as possible.

My second tiny fear had to do with what would occur should I require some assistance and I were the only human within a twenty-mile radius who spoke any English, and the sun was fading fast in the west.

This thought gave me further impetus to learn the Korean language as quickly as possible. And it wasn't long before some of the reporters began asking me where a certain town was located, and the interrogators began speaking to me in rudimentary Korean.

As mentioned earlier, the fact that so many opportunities had been open to me was because I prepared myself for these eventualities. Rarely do opportunities simply plop down on your lap; no, you must latch onto the brass ring as it flies past at a pretty good clip or else be left sucking sea breezes.

The two things I chose to do to further my education – the map and learning the Korean language – unwittingly prepared me for my next great opportunity for advancement. And I must say, for the most interesting period of my young life. What an adventure! The experiences were priceless.

The colonel who commanded the 502 was quite popular with his men. The post, like the *Stars & Stripes* compound, was relatively small in size. One could sail a flat rock from one side of the compound to the other with relative ease, and at any one time there were likely no more than forty soldiers on post, including the six or seven prisoner interrogators.

As there was not any great degree of supervision required of the interrogators – no one knew the job better than did they – the colonel remained inside his office a good part of the work day.

I knew the colonel as well as did any of the *Stars & Stripes* reporters. He was quite accessible and if he were not in his office we could find him over at the mess hall having coffee with some of the men of the 502 or the reporters from the *Stars & Stripes*. In addition he took his meals in the mess hall with us, so he had a good opportunity to observe the men.

I had been at the *Stars & Stripes* for about thirteen months, going where I wanted to go, when I wanted to go and coming back whenever I pleased. About once a month the thin-skinned North Koreans or Chinese would get their feathers ruffled over some real or perceived offense committed by one or two of Captain Neely's M.P.s, and I would be summoned to Panmunjom to gather information to write my story. There is, and was, no doubt in my mind that three-fourths of the communists' complaints against the American M.P.s held truth. Captain Neely's men just didn't give a damn. Good for them.

I had been the feature writer for about thirteen months when at breakfast one morning the 502 colonel finished eating and passed by my table on the way to his office, which happened to be located in the same building as was the mess hall.

The colonel paused and we exchanged greetings. "Are you in a hurry to get somewhere this morning Provost?"

"No sir, colonel. What can I do for you?"

"I've got an opportunity you might just be interested in. Stop by the office after breakfast and we can discuss it."

"Thanks colonel. I'll be right there," I said.

"We have a problem here at the 502 that you might be able to help us with," he said gesturing toward the visitor's chair across the desk. I sat but decided to let him have the first word.

"You have observed of course that a few Korean men dressed in civilian clothes visit my office on a fairly regular basis."

"Yes sir I have," I replied.

"This is because this compound, although under the control of the U.S. Army, is also home to the Korean army's counterintelligence command."

"So the Korean army gets what you get," I added nodding my head.

"In fact there are three persons inside the interrogation room at all times; the prisoner, the Korean Army interrogator, and the U.S. Army interrogator.

"Who actually interrogates the prisoner?" I asked.

"Both the Korean and the American interrogators. However anyone would be foolish if he believed that an American who has studied Korean for 47 weeks could boast of being as fluent as a native Korean, don't you agree?" he said.

"Most assuredly," I responded.

"So what we do is to take the top ten or twelve students from the graduates of the Defense Language Institute and send them to the U.S. Army Intelligence Center located in Baltimore, Maryland, to take the eight-week course in Prisoner Interrogation."

"So how long does it take the American prisoner interrogator, sitting in a room with a South Korean prisoner interrogator and a North Korean prisoner, to be able to interrogate a prisoner on his own?"

"I would say no longer than two-to-three months," responded the colonel.

Suddenly it came to me that the good colonel was about to offer me a job.

And he did. Right then and there.

"Another thing that impresses me is that apparently, from what my interrogators tell me, you have memorized the road map of Korea. And I've never seen anyone do that before."

"It wasn't all that difficult really. Like any other *splinter skill*, once you focus all your time on that single subject it becomes easier to learn. And memorizing the road map assured me that I'd never again get lost."

"Knowing by heart the roadmap of Korea is really quite an asset to the interrogators.

This means that you don't have to consult a road map every time you need to ask a prisoner the location of such-and-such a town, or how long it took him to drive from Sokcho to Taegu. If he states it took him eight hours to make the trip, you should be able to determine whether he is telling the truth by knowing from memory whether the drive took eight hours or sixteen hours."

"In addition to towns and distances, I also know which roads become impassable during heavy rains," I said. I related to the colonel my near-disaster when following the Honest John Rocket convoy from Chunchon.

"Same with bridges and pole-barges," I added. "The prisoner might tell you he drove from Wonsan to Pusan. However, if the map shows this, and the road crosses a river, there is a 50-50 chance there was no bridge across the river and that he and his vehicle could only have crossed the river on a pole-barge. And I know the location of every pole-barge crossing in South Korea. Just look for a wide river."

At this point the colonel's demeanor led me to believe what I sensed was a certainty about the prospective job offer. The dead giveaway was when he reached over and lifted a brown personnel folder off the corner of his desk. He placed the folder on the desk and opened it.

"The captain over at the *Stars & Stripes* office around the corner loaned me your file, which is very impressive. You must know someone in the FBI."

"How is this, sir?" I asked innocently.

"Provost, I don't know how you pulled this off, but your file indicates that at the time you joined the army you already possessed a Top Secret Security Clearance."

"That is correct sir."

"And security clearances are only issued by the FBI, not the U.S. Army."

"I understand, sir."

If the colonel's two comments were intended to elicit some explanation from me, in this regard they failed. I had vowed to myself that I would never explain the circumstances to anyone. And anyone included the nice colonel.

Apparently realizing I had no intention of offering an explanation, he picked up the file, studied it for a few moments in silence, then put it down.

"Provost your tour of duty here in Korea ends in two months. According to your C.O.

(Commanding Officer), they would be happy if you extended your tour as the feature writer, but you may be looking for something a little more challenging. If so, I have an offer to make. You can take it or leave it, and no hard feelings should you decline the offer."

"Could you explain it to me in a nutshell, sir?" An outline of the offer follows.

What Army Intelligence needed in Korea were a few (really) good prisoner interrogators.

Like for example someone who had been studying Korean on his own for the past year.

Like for example someone who had memorized the road map of Korea and knew the geography of the country like the back of his hand.

Like for example someone who already possessed a Top Secret Security Clearance that naturally would be required of any prisoner interrogator.

Like for example, Spec-4 Al Provost.

So how do we go about doing this? If I happened to be interested, that is.

I had been in the army nearly eighteen months of a 36-month enlistment. To prepare myself to return to Seoul as a prisoner interrogator I had to:

Wait two months for the next Korean language class to begin at the Defense Language Institute, located in the coastal tourist town of Monterey, California.

Attend the 47-week language course. Classes were taught six hours per day, five days per week, with homework to do every night.

Following graduation from the Defense Language Institute, travel from Monterey,

California to the U.S. Army Intelligence Center, located in Baltimore, Maryland, to undergo the 8-week course in Prisoner Interrogation before returning to Seoul, Korea as a prisoner interrogator, interrogating North Korean espionage agents captured by the South Korean army while attempting to infiltrate into South Korea along the craggy East Sea coastline.

The language course of 47 weeks, plus the two-month wait time for the next class to begin, plus the 8-week prisoner interrogation course at Ft. Holabird in Baltimore, Maryland, plus a month's leave would mean that I would come to the end of my three-year enlistment before I ever returned to Korea. So what do we do about this, I asked the colonel.

I knew there had to be an answer. After four and a half years of wearing "army green" I learned there are no unsolvable problems as far as the U.S. Army is concerned. So I wasn't worried.

The army makes allowances for these odd situations, he replied. First I would receive an early discharge from my 36-month enlistment. The following day I would re-enlist in the army for another 36-month tour. So when I was discharged for the second time I would have spent a total of four years and four months in the U.S. Army. So I quickly weighed the extra sixteen months against having an opportunity to experience the world of prisoner interrogation. Why I'd make that trade-off any day under God's bright sun.

"I want to thank you for this opportunity," I told the colonel. "I suppose I'm ready to start anytime."

Ten days later the 502 colonel met me at breakfast over at the 502 mess hall.

"Provost, stop by Eighth Army Personnel down at Yongsan. Any time today will be fine."

At the huge personnel center the personnel officer and I went through the motions of receiving the Honorable Discharge document. He gave me a copy of the document for my records.

"Now come back tomorrow and we'll go through the re-enlistment ceremony," he said.

"Could we just do it all today and save myself a trip?" I asked.

"I'd like to be able to help," he said. "However the records would show that you re-enlisted on the same day you received an Honorable Discharge; and for whatever reason we were told not to do it this way."

So I returned the following morning, re-enlisted for three years, then returned to the *Stars & Stripes* and began setting my affairs in order in preparation to leave Korea.

The Army Language School
AKA The Defense Language Institute
Monterey, California

I arrived at the United States Army Language School (ALS) in June 1963, and completed the 47-week Korean Language course. Even at the time, I sensed ALS to be a misnomer not reflecting the true mission of the school. A goodly percentage of ALS students were from the U.S. Navy, Air Force, Marine Corps, as well as the "suits," as we called those students from the FBI, CIA, NSA and a few other alphabet-soup federal agencies. The Presidio of Monterey however was considered to be a U.S. Army installation and was under the operational control of the U.S. Army.

The Coat of Arms on the front cover of our textbooks read *ARMY LANGUAGE SCHOOL*. The following was printed on the first page of the textbook: "A total of twenty-eight foreign languages are taught at the school."

The Korean language textbooks I used were published in May 1959. They were revised in January 1961, and reprinted in September 1962.

The address of the language school, as printed on the bottom of the first page was asfollows:

United States Army Language School
Presidio of Monterey, California

Based on this information then, I arrived at the Army Language School nine months after the textbooks were reprinted in September 1962. Years later the name of the school was changed to Defense Language Institute-West Coast Campus (DLI-WC) to more accurately define its mission. However the Institute remained under the operational control of the U.S. Army.

Diversity became abundantly clear the moment I entered the two story, all-brick college classrooms on the first day of class. The school was built on the grounds of the Presidio of Monterey. There were two roughly-speaking "Companies," denoted Company A and Company B.

Company A had been constructed atop the Presidio. It consisted of the two-story all brick modern dormitory where students lived two to a room, and a two-story all-brick building housing classrooms. Company A was referred to as *the school on top of the hill.*

Company B was referred to as *the school at the bottom of the hill.* And the wooden barracks and wooden classroom building indeed had been constructed at the very bottom of the steep hill.

I had arrived at the small commuter airport near Monterey two days before the beginning of classes, and had taken a taxi to the Company A office that was located on the ground floor of the large two-story brick building. I signed in using a copy of my orders, and was given a key to a room located on the second floor. I noted that two men were assigned to a room.

Following a lively supper I stopped by the wall corkboard down the hall to find the name of the U.S. Army soldier who was supposed to be my roommate. I then returned to my room to discover that he had not yet arrived.

On the way to my room I passed by several army corporals carrying on a conversation in the hall. I asked whether any of them knew my roommate.

"I know him," said one soldier. "But he decided not to enroll. He wanted to study Spanish but they signed him up for the Chinese class, and he said no way in hell would he study Chinese. Would you?"

Probably not, I thought but did not say. I thanked the men and continued on down the hall. If anyone discovered I really did not have a roommate, he surely wouldn't get this information from me.

And apparently my silence paid big dividends. Forty-seven weeks later on the date of our graduation there were perhaps a half dozen of us who still did not have roommates. We had agreed to keep our mouth shut.

The following day, that was the day before classes started, the Company A students gathered in the large auditorium at the bottom of the hill, where we learned the rules of the Army Language School.

The commandant of the Presidio was a U.S. Army colonel. The civilian students were in attendance also, because everyone needed to know the operation of the school.

The first thing the colonel said was for the army students who were at the time wearing the summer (khaki) uniforms, to store these uniforms away inside their footlockers, and for the next year to wear only the winter (olive drab) uniforms. The reason: The moderate temperatures of Monterey made it too cool to wear the summer uniform, even during the summer months.

The majority of languages were 47-week courses. The exceptions were the Romance languages. Spanish, German, French, Italian and a few others were only 6-month courses, for obvious reasons.

The Southeast Asian, Oriental and Far Eastern languages, including Chinese, Japanese and Korean, as well as Vietnamese, Burmese, Laotian, Thai and Cambodian, were taught on the Company A campus at the top of the hill.

The Slavic, Middle Eastern and Eastern European languages, including Norwegian, Danish, Swedish, German, Polish, Russian and Czechoslovakian among others, were taught on the Company B campus at the bottom of the hill.

Classes were in session six hours per day, five days per week. There were no classes on the weekend.

In most instances there were thirty students per class, broken down into three classrooms of ten students each.

The faculty was second to none. Each instructor must have been a college professor in his or her native country. For each class three classrooms were required. Thus each course required a department head and three instructors, one for each of three classrooms.

When classes started on the day following the assembly, the breakdown of which ten students were assigned to which classroom was entirely arbitrary.

We were tested daily, in translation, grammar and listening comprehension. The first part of each lesson involved a dialogue between two students. Each student had to memorize both halves of the conversation.

When class started at 9:00 a.m. the first two students stood at the front of the classroom *without the textbook*. The students were denoted Student A and Student B. They went through the conversation.

After finishing the dialogue the two students changed sides, whereupon Student A played Student B's part and vice versa.

The daily translation tests were difficult. What was needed to be translated in writing was not written on a sheet of paper or even on the chalkboard. Each student took out a clean sheet of notebook paper and placed it on the desk before him.

The instructor read aloud *twice only* the sentence, in English. The students had one minute to write down the translation in Korean. A request from a student for the instructor to repeat the sentence *a third time* in English was met with a shake of the instructor's head. Which in just about any language means *No*.

On the first day of class following the day of the assembly, we thirty students were milling about in the hall awaiting who we learned was Professor Kim, the head of the Korean Department, when I heard one of the Marines voice the following complaint.

"I don't know what I'm doing here. I certainly didn't sign up for this. And I sure as hell don't want to go to Korea."

This unexpected – to me at least – comment caught the attention of a second Marine who offered up a reasonable explanation for the first Marine's presence:

"When I received my orders to report here, I asked the clerk in personnel the same question. He said the Marines had to fill their quota. I know I don't want to be here, but we have to go where we're told to go."

Suddenly I had reservations about what I had gotten myself into. And at my first opportunity I would pass my concerns by Professor Kim.

I have found from experience dating back to my teenage years that if you are polite, helpful and appreciative, you'd be amazed at how far out of their way that people will go to lend you a helping hand.

So on a coffee break the following morning I cornered Professor Kim and asked whether I could speak to him after classes ended for the day. And to ensure I received a positive response from the rotund, smooth-skinned professor I spoke to him in fluent Korean. He broke out in a grin.

When I met him after class, I related to him my concerns that I might end up in a class with several students who had no interest in being at the Army Language School. So I was relieved at his explanation, as follows:

The administration recognized such concerns. So following the first four weeks of class the top ten students, grade-wise, were assigned to Room A, the second ten to Room B and the ten students with the lowest grades were placed in Room C. The staff agreed this was the most equitable method of placing students.

Because I had studied Korean for nearly a year on my own, I did my homework at night, then studied the advance lessons. When classes began each student received all the textbooks he would require for the entire course.

In 1963 audiotapes were in their infancy. Thus each student also received a recording machine and spools of *wire*. These were known as "wire recorders," and the quality of the sound was remarkably good. By listening to these wire recordings at night we could refine our pronunciation for class the following day.

U.S. Army students all lived in the large two-story dormitory. All students attended class as follows: Classes were in session from 9:00 a.m. until noon. This was followed by the lunch period from noon until 2:00 p.m. Afternoon classes were in session from 2:00 p.m. until 5:00 p.m.

This schedule was followed Monday-Friday. There were no classes on the weekend. We U.S. Army students "fell out" for inspection at 9:00 a.m. Saturday, which lasted every bit of fifteen minutes. We were on our own for the remainder of the weekend.

In 1963 Monterey, California was a relatively small and quiet tourist town. The town had been built on the ocean, and there were plenty of quiet bars along U.S. 1 and the wide Cannery Row of John Steinbeck fame.

There was a side entrance to Company A atop the hill that was open only during the day.

The gate was locked at 5:00 p.m. However if we walked out of this entrance and continued three blocks on down the hill we were on busy U.S. 1. And best of all there was no curfew, even during the week.

Mixed in with the military students were a goodly number of men and women who lived off-campus and wore civilian clothes. We were told these students were attached to one of several U.S. government agencies, mainly the FBI, CIA and the NSA. We were also cautioned not to pry into the affairs of these civilians.

The Arrogant Colonel

I would like to report that my year spent studying Korean at the Defense Language Institute had been a raving success. However this had not been the case. Most of the ten students assigned to the slower Classroom C were in the same sorry situation as were the Marines mentioned just above, who had not signed up to attend the language school. You can lead a horse to water, etcetera etcetera…

These soldiers had been caught up in the military's *quota system*, that mandated that because there were spaces in each class for thirty students, and there were only twenty students available who wanted to be there, the other ten spaces would be filled by soldiers who had scored high on the language aptitude tests administered by the military.

And the U.S. Army had had years of experience with such situations. Recall the *Draft?* Same difference.

Confine ten soldiers in an enclosed space, ten soldiers who did not ask to be there, and expect these ten soldiers to sit quietly and learn a strange, very difficult language is a recipe for certain disaster.

Those ten soldiers and Marines laughed and joked and carried on throughout the six hours of class each day, until their Korean instructor, in utter frustration complained to the colonel, the highest-ranking officer among our class of thirty students. And how did the colonel take care of the problem?

He simply walked down to Classroom A and called me out into the hall. Yes, me.

"Provost, the instructor in Room C is having a discipline problem in that room."

"How does that involve me, sir?" I asked.

"I want you to grab your books and move down to Room C. Just make sure you hold down the noise level and see that those men do what the instructor tells them to do."

"For how long do I have to do this?"

"The rest of the school year. It's a permanent change."

The hell you say colonel, thought I, having decided to plead my case.

"But sir, I'm only a Spec-4. At least half of the ten students outrank me, and three of the ten are Marines and have nothing to do with me."

"But *I* have something to do with you, Provost. I'm the ranking officer here, and I've just given you a direct order. Now pick up your books, go down to Classroom C and take care of the problem."

I did as ordered, and spent the rest of the day sitting in Classroom C. No way in hell was I going to obey the arrogant colonel's orders. I had made my decision before classes ended for the day.

The Commandant of the Presidio of Monterey was a colonel also. The colonel who ordered me to move to Classroom C *was merely a student* at the Army Language School. He had nothing to do with assigning students to classrooms. Such assignments were solely under the control of the Commandant.

Suspecting this to be the case, at 8:00 a.m. the following day I reported to the Office of the Commandant. The young female corporal seated at the desk in the outer office asked me whether I had an appointment to see the Commandant.

"No, I do not have an appointment, Corporal. However it is a matter of extreme urgency, and I'll just sit out here and wait for him. If you need to pull my personnel file, my name is Alton L. Provost and my serial number is RA 13732036."

I waited as the corporal pulled my file from the file room, carried it into the colonel's office and closed the door. The reason the corporal and the colonel remained behind the closed office door likely had something to do with my Top Secret Security Clearance. It caused everyone to hesitate.

Finally the office door opened and the corporal asked me to enter. Then she closed the door on her way to the receptionist's desk in the outer office.

Before I could salute the colonel, he waved me to the visitor's chair across the desk.

"Provost, it appears from your file that you are to complete the Korean course, then go to Ft. Holabird for the Prisoner Interrogation Course and from there back to the 502nd Military Intelligence Battalion in Seoul. Is this correct, son?"

"Yes sir, this is correct."

"I see from your record that you already have a Top Secret Security Clearance. How long have you had this clearance? I ask because you appear to be a bit young to already have a Top Secret Security Clearance."

"I graduated from college on May 15, 1961. Two weeks later the FBI gave me the Top Secret Clearance."

"Your personnel file shows that you enlisted in the army on June 30, 1961. So according to the record, at the time you enlisted you already had a Top Secret Security Clearance. Is this correct?"

"Yes sir, it is."

What ensued was a very long pause, as though the colonel were deciding whether to delve into this unusual set of circumstances, or simply let well enough alone. He opted for the latter course.

"Based on your record Provost, it is readily apparent that Army Intelligence wants you back in Seoul as soon as possible. And I'm not one to stand in your way. So how can I help you?"

It took less than five minutes to state the facts and the problem in clear and succinct terms, while the colonel nodded his head as though he had encountered this same situation more than once in the past.

"This problem has occurred enough times that the army has toyed with the idea of making every student here wear civilian clothes. But as long as the soldiers wear uniforms the higher ranking officers believe they have the authority to order around the enlisted men."

"I understand, sir," I said.

"But he *doesn't*. The colonel was out of line in ordering you to change classrooms, and I won't allow this to happen."

"What should I do, sir?"

"For today you just stay away from the classrooms. We wouldn't want to cause the colonel any embarrassment. Later this morning I'll have one of my officers go to the classroom and explain to the colonel that any discipline problems or class placement problems will be handled *by the army* and not by a student regardless of his rank."

"Sir, I hope I have not caused you any problems by complaining."

"To the contrary, Provost. In my push to have everyone attending the Army Language School wear civilian clothes, I can use your case as a specific example in stating my position."

I thanked the commandant and the female corporal, then exited the headquarters building. There was a well-stocked foreign language library on campus, so I spent the day reading ancient Korean history.

The following morning when classes began at 9:00 o'clock, I walked into Classroom A and took my usual seat. The day's classes proceeded as normal, except when the students started their little between-class coffee break I made sure I was as far away as possible from the colonel. And apparently he knew better than retaliate against me because I never had any problems with him after that day.

At the end of the 47-week course the thirty of us students as a group went by bus up north of Monterey to the foreign language testing center at Ft. Ord, for our final exams. And I am serious when I make the following observation: Out of the ten students in Classroom C (the slower students), at least eight of the ten could not translate "I need to go to the bathroom," in Korean. After 47 weeks of instruction.

What a waste.

Learning the Difficult Korean Language

Ample evidence exists that Korean is one of the most difficult languages to learn at the Defense Language Institute. *The Miami Herald*, Wed., Feb. 8, 1967 issue, carried the following story on page 18-A.

"The Director here is Army Col. Richard L. Long. Long is a student of languages. He can talk to you about any language and in fact speaks many of the 27 tongues taught at this rather unique school."

The teaching staff consists of 500 language instructors, who teach 2,600 students. The learning week is 30 hours.

The toughest language to learn, in Long's view, is Korean.

"It's far more difficult to learn, for example, than either Chinese or Russian. The Russian language is more logical. Once you pick up a few words, the others seem to fall into place. It isn't so with Korean. Most students here master Russian or Chinese in nine to 12 months, but it takes many of them at least 18 months to figure out Korean."

I fully agree with Col. Long's take concerning the difficulty of learning languages. I find the study of languages fascinating and challenging.

Using the learning format perfected at the Defense Language Institute, I have studied the following seven languages a minimum of two years: Arabic, Russian, Japanese, Spanish, Italian, French and Korean. Far and away the most difficult to learn has been Korean. An undertaking definitely not for the faint of heart.

Quality of Instruction – Monterey and Baltimore

From 1957 to 1961 I studied Physics and Mathematics at Berry College, earning my undergraduate degree (B.S. Physics-Mathematics).

Following my Honorable Discharge from the U.S. Army in November 1965 I earned a doctorate in Optometry (O.D.) from the University of Houston in 1972, and in 1980 a doctorate in Law (Juris Doctor) from Nova Southeastern University College of Law.

Thus after four years of undergraduate school and another eight years in graduate school, I'm pleased to say that scholastically-speaking I've done quite well.

Because of this I have tended to equate – either fairly or not – my academic success with *how well I was taught* by these professors. And I laud them all for preparing me to excel in my studies.

Likewise I have utilized this same criteria in assessing the quality of education I received at the Defense Language Institute for nearly a year and at the U.S. Army Intelligence Center for eight weeks.

At both schools the instructors were always well-prepared, eager to explain in greater detail if we students did not understand a point, and encouraged us in our learning. I am indebted to these educators for their professionalism.

In order to avoid any redundancies in the telling of my story, I will cut short any explanation of the material taught at Ft. Holabird and will discuss this as part of my actual experiences as the youngest prisoner interrogator at Company A, 502 Military Intelligence Battalion, Seoul, Korea in 1964-1965.

I was to discover from the veteran interrogator who had picked me up at Kimpo Airport upon my arrival, and others, that the half-dozen interrogators stationed at the 502 constituted a close-knit fraternity from whom I was to learn my craft. They were excellent teachers.

The Assassination of President Kennedy

We were expected to be seated inside our classrooms promptly for the beginning of the morning class and the afternoon session. In order to allow for personal business we were given a two-hour lunch break from 12:00 noon to 2:00 p.m. each day.

When classes let out at 12:00 noon we usually strolled from the classroom building across the large grassy area to the dormitory building that also housed the kitchen and spacious mess hall.

Lunch rarely ever took longer than a half hour, leaving an hour and a half of free time before classes resumed at 2:00 p.m.

The coffee shop was situated in a small building located approximately midway between the classrooms and the dormitory-mess hall. We often drifted over from the mess hall, stopping by for a soft drink or cup of coffee, to read the day's San Francisco *Chronicle and shoot the breeze* about world events and baseball scores.

While a student at Berry College (1957-1961) I had worked in the college Print Shop as a Linotype operator and proofreader, where I ran smack-dab into the *Curse of the Proofreader.*

To be a good proofreader one must learn to read every single solitary word of the material he is *proofing*, as it is called. Do this for a year or two and you will find yourself for the remainder of your life, reading every store sign, magazine headline and roadside billboard that happens to fall within your line of sight. Even down to the printing on the wrapping of a candy bar.

Thus after reading the daily issue of the San Francisco *Chronicle* inside the coffee shop on the Army Language School campus for about two months, I reached the following frustrating and disappointing conclusion:

The most poorly-written, error-filled (grammar, spelling and punctuation) big-city daily I had ever read was hands-down the "esteemed" San Francisco *Chronicle*. The only consistent non-quality aspect of the newspaper was its mediocrity. After two months I gave up and never again read the newspaper.

I became an observer of human nature the day I arrived at Oxford Orphanage at the age of seven on February 15, 1947. Even then I could spot a phony at twenty paces just by listening to him speak for five minutes…or less.

And so it was with John F. Kennedy, who became the 35th President of the United States in January 1961, four months before I graduated from Berry College on May 15, 1961.

By the time of his taking the oath of office John F. Kennedy, with the help of the press and Hollywood celebrities, had elevated himself to the status of a revered statesman. Poppycock!

And because of Kennedy's apparent popularity with the press, I never read any unflattering account of anything he ever said or did. I observed however, following my arrival in Korea in January 1962, a year following his much-publicized inauguration in January 1961, that I very rarely heard the president's name even mentioned, in any context.

Recall that the *Stars & Stripes* was a daily newspaper. It was just as thick as any big-city daily. And it was in no sense of the word a *military* newspaper. The first section was devoted to United States and international news. There was a large sports and entertainment section. There was no section devoted solely to military news; rather stories containing my byline were interspersed among the other sections.

As I recall however, the one salient fact that stood out clearly in my mind was the dearth of news articles featuring John F. Kennedy, President of the United States.

By August of 1963 President Kennedy was convinced that he needed to move politically closer to Martin Luther King's civil rights movement. However if he drifted too far to the left he chanced incurring the wrath of the well-entrenched *silent majority* of white male voters. Some of these sentiments had already surfaced by late September 1963.

The Morning of November 22, 1963

On the morning of November 22, 1963 we attended classes from 9:00 a.m.-12:00 noon. Then we meandered from the classroom building across the expansive and well-kept field to the mess hall, where we enjoyed our usual leisurely lunch.

At approximately 12:30 p.m. several small groups of us left the mess hall and wandered on over to the coffee shop. I later recalled ordering a bottled Coke (metal soft drink cans were still in their infancy) and a Baby Ruth candy bar. I drank the Coke but decided to save the candy bar for a between-class snack.

When I exited the coffee shop I was walking between two small groups of students in the direction of the classroom building. Suddenly I heard the voice of a student as he followed a group out the door.

"Did you all hear that? Kennedy's been shot." A tone of neither shock nor surprise.

I recall at that moment pausing, as though expecting to get some directions as to what we should do, from the student who had just informed us of the shooting.

However no instructions were forthcoming. The students continued walking toward the classroom building, so I followed the group. In an act that I considered strange at the moment, none of the group of students even asked whether Kennedy had been assassinated, or whether the shooter had been apprehended.

I got the distinct impression that as a group of fifteen or more, none seemed to even care what had befallen the president.

When we reached the classroom building, seemingly still in no hurry to spread what I thought should have been devastating, unforgettable news, we observed small groups of students carrying on quiet conversations, but on a myriad of topics, only some of which dealt with one of the most important events of the Twentieth Century.

The beginning and ending of classes were controlled by a not very loud buzzer. Between classes students had ample time to get a cup of coffee and smoke a cigarette before the next buzzer sounded.

By listening to various conversations being carried out between classes I came away with the very distinct impression that the assassination of the President of the United States ranked right alongside reading the box score of a baseball game between two cellar-dwelling semi-pro baseball teams.

What's more, I noticed that I myself had not been terribly impressed with this momentous event.

Some years later an acquaintance asked me: "Do you recall what you were doing the day President Kennedy was shot?"

"Yes I do. I was a student at the Defense Language Institute in Monterey, California. A group of us had just finished eating lunch and we were walking across the big lawn on our way to the classroom."

"What did you do when you heard the news?"

"I just continued walking."

"Did they cut classes short for the day?"

"No. Why should they have cut classes short?"

"Well did they cancel classes for the following day?"

"No. Why should they have cancelled classes?"

I was in the U.S. Army for nearly four and a half years. The U.S. Army is controlled by rank. In this situation the Commandant of the Presidio apparently believed he did not possess the authority to either cut classes short or cancel the following day's classes.

Nevertheless I have always thought these circumstances odd, even though it seemed to be common knowledge that President Kennedy had not been a fan of the U.S. military. The lesson: Not all momentous historical events come with a logical explanation. This one did not.

Chapter 12

◇◇◇◇◇

U.S. Army Intelligence Center
Ft. Holabird, Maryland – 1964

After graduating from the 47-week Korean Language Course at the Army Language School at the top of my class of thirty students, following a 10-day leave I reported to the U.S. Army Intelligence Center, located in Baltimore, Maryland, to undergo the eight-week course in Prisoner Interrogation Theory and Practice.

Although my ultimate goal was to return to Korea as a prisoner interrogator, instruction at Ft. Holabird was not geared to a specific language. And just as at the Army Language School, all the major branches of the service were represented at the Intelligence Center.

Incorporated into the lectures and instruction on the various techniques of prisoner interrogation was the associated course dealing with the interpretation of aerial photographs taken by CIA pilots flying the U-2 reconnaissance aircraft at 60,000 feet.

After completing the eight-week prisoner interrogation and aerial photograph interpretation course and being stationed at Company A, 502 Military Intelligence Battalion in Seoul, I learned the importance of my job when the colonel commanding the 502 informed me of the pivotal role our unit played in counterintelligence in Korea.

"Of all the intelligence we gather on North Korea," he said, "ninety percent comes from our interrogation of captured North Korean espionage agents and ten percent comes from the U-2 aerial photographs."

When I arrived at Ft. Holabird following graduating at the top of my Korean Language class at the Army Language School, I expected to see ten or possibly more of these language graduates taking the prisoner interrogation course with me at Ft. Holabird. However this was not to be.

Of the thirty Korean language students, only four attended the Prisoner Interrogation Course at Ft. Holabird with me.

By the same token, near the end of the eight-week course at Ft. Holabird, I checked the barracks bulletin board and discovered that I was the only one of the five of us who had been assigned to the 502 in Seoul.

Initially I was puzzled by this turn of events. However a few questions to the staff at Ft. Holabird enabled me to figure it out. And it made logical sense. Attrition was the key, said the officer.

At the time I arrived at the Defense Language Institute in Monterey, California in 1963, more likely than not the projected need for Korean-speaking prisoner interrogators a year later would be no more than five.

So just because a soldier believed he could learn the language and become proficient within 47 weeks, there were several logical reasons why this might not occur. This fact then required that there be a beginning "pool" of wannabe Korean linguists. They would begin with a pool of thirty hoping that at least five would survive the course at the language school and come away with any degree of fluency.

So now we send the surviving five Korean linguists to Ft. Holabird, Maryland, hoping that four out of five not only would complete the eight-week course in prisoner interrogation but would actually enjoy the challenge.

The second consideration is, what would occur if five men passed the language course *and* the prisoner interrogation course and expected to go from Ft. Holabird to Seoul, Korea and the 502 Military Intelligence Battalion, except that the 502 *needed only one* prisoner interrogator? It was a guessing game, a crap shoot for certain.

This scenario is precisely what occurred in my case, as I discovered upon my arrival at Kimpo Airport south of Seoul in the autumn of 1964.

One of the interrogators was waiting inside the terminal when the plane landed. He welcomed me to Korea and after collecting my duffel bag we climbed into his Jeep and headed north toward Seoul.

"Are any of the other guys from Ft. Holabird here yet?" I asked by way of making conversation.

"You're the only one," he replied.

"I suppose the others will be arriving in a day or two?" I asked expectantly.

"No Provost, it's just you. We were short only one interrogator and now that you are here we've got all we need."

The drive from Kimpo Airport to Seoul took longer than an hour. My driver and I carried on a lengthy conversation – in Korean – beginning the moment we met inside the terminal.

"Your Korean is a lot better than mine," I said in English, laughing as I spoke. "You speak like a native."

"Well I should," he said in English. "I've been married to a Korean woman for ten years, so I end up speaking Korean most of the time."

We chatted in English for awhile, small talk about family and such. I sensed he wanted to change the subject but didn't know how. Finally he spoke.

"The colonel told us you were at the *Stars & Stripes* before you went to the Army Language School, and that you know Korea better than do most Americans. How is this?"

"Well I was the newspaper's feature writer for fifteen months. I was assigned my own Jeep and allowed to roam at will throughout Korea," I answered.

"I had a map but was afraid I might misplace it one day. So I made it my mission to memorize every road and town in the country, including mileage between towns. And I did the same with North Korea."

"This will really come in handy when you begin analyzing the mission of the communist agents and their minders," the driver said. "The first information we need from a captured agent is his destination in South Korea and the identity of the agents waiting in their safehouses. In tracing the agent's route I and the other interrogators must have the map spread out on the table. However you should be able to track his route and immediately tell whether or not he is lying."

I figured I could ask this interrogator at least thirty pertinent prisoner interrogation questions during our drive from Kimpo Airport to the 502, located in the Yungdung-po district of Seoul. However he suddenly realized he was out of bounds in this revealing conversation.

"I suppose I'd better let you save your questions for the colonel," he said. "I wouldn't want to tell you one thing and have him tell you something different. You understand I'm sure."

"You're correct," I responded. And then I recalled the officer who had recruited me.

"By the way, is Col. Bradley (not his real name) still commanding the 502?" I asked.

"Yes he is. The colonel is one of the good guys. Stays out of the interrogators' way and lets us do our job. But he'll be rotating stateside in about six months."

"Do the guys from the *Stars & Stripes* still take their meals with you at the 502?"

"No they don't. A few months ago the army moved their office to the building on Yongsan compound that houses the Eighth Army Information Office of Col. Creel."

"Did anyone give a reason for the move?"

"We heard that the reporters had too much freedom. Now they bunk in the barracks on Yongsan, eat at the main mess hall and have to sign out a Jeep in the morning and sign it back in before 6:00 p.m."

"Boy, those reporters must really be upset. I never would have taken the job as feature writer if I had all the restrictions that these guys now have."

We made small talk for awhile until I recalled the white Kaopectate-like substance in the bottles the interrogators carried with them everywhere they went.

"How many of the interrogators have ulcers?" I asked. "When I was here with the *Stars & Stripes* we took our meals with the guys at the 502, and it seemed like all the interrogators carried the small bottle of chalky liquid around with them."

"The colonel will go over the pros and cons of being a prisoner interrogator. Most of us make it to the end of our tour in one piece, both physically and psychologically. You'll see the reason that every man who becomes a prisoner interrogator must first attend the eight-week course at Ft. Holabird. Some don't complete the course."

On Becoming a Prisoner Interrogator
U.S. Army Intelligence Center Ft. Holabird, Maryland

In 1963 there existed one cast-in-stone rule concerning the United States Army: It had its own way of doing things. Period.

An excellent example of this tenet was the Prisoner Interrogation Course at Ft. Holabird. The faculty consisted of a half dozen or so officers, and my eight weeks of training flashed before me as the driver of the Jeep sped down the road from Kimpo Airport late on the day of my arrival in Korea.

The major in charge of our class had made a few things clear on the first day of lectures.

"Take every preconceived notion you have about the role of a prisoner interrogator, including those from old World War II spy movies, and toss them into a trash can," he began.

"A good psychologist is the best prisoner interrogator, and our goal is to produce a class of good psychologists," he explained further. "We're giving you the tools to work with. The interrogators at the post you're headed for will fill in the blanks, and you'll be glad you had these eight-weeks' head start.

The first few days of class were devoted to the thoughts going through the prisoner's mind prior to the first interrogation session.

"You the interrogator are studying the prisoner's demeanor at that first meeting. But bear in mind that at that same encounter the prisoner is also studying *your* demeanor," cautioned the colonel.

"So you must leave your emotions outside the interrogation room before you even open that door. You can never exhibit signs of surprise, displeasure, disappointment, disgust or impatience. And never ever show frustration."

"Sir, I believe you are describing a good poker player, is this correct?" quipped one of the students.

"And that's about the best analogy I can think of," said the course instructor. "What you need to develop is a good poker face. And tomorrow we'll start play-acting using members of the faculty."

The officer-instructor went on to remind us that likely before the eight-week course ended, several of us would find that we simply were not cut out to be prisoner interrogators. If this occurred we were to quietly inform the instructor.

The eight-week course began with a class of thirty students, same as the standard course at the Defense Language Institute. However whereas the language class of thirty was further divided into three rooms of ten students each for efficiency in learning, at Ft. Holabird the thirty students assembled in a single classroom, then moved to different areas of the large classroom for demonstrations and role-playing.

And the officer-instructor proved true to his prediction. By the end of Week No. 5 our beginning class of thirty had dwindled to twenty-one, and we jokingly referred to ourselves as the "survivors."

And of these survivors, pride was the only thing that kept some in the program. In our last week of class we twenty-one held a little "graduation party" in the Enlisted Men's Club at Ft. Holabird. By then we had received orders giving our next posting, at which time I found that I was the only linguist assigned to the 502 Military Intelligence Battalion in Seoul.

The Fascinating Field of Aerial Photography

In addition to delving meticulously into various techniques of prisoner interrogation, in the third week we were introduced to the art of interpreting aerial photographs.

"In nearly every interrogation you will need to know the route the prisoner took in arriving at the point on the map where he was captured," explained the instructor. "And in the real world the U-2 spy plane pilots can give you nearly next-day service on the aerial photographs you require. And that's about as close to *real time* as we can get."

The aerial photograph is laid out under clear glass on a long table, and a powerful magnifying glass is placed on a stand above the glass. In 1963 the quality of the photographs we studied at Baltimore was remarkable and state-of-the-art.

The aerial photograph is one of the most useful tools in determining whether the prisoner is telling the truth concerning things located or not located in a certain part of town, or the path the prisoner took to arrive at his destination. He believes he can afford to lie because you would have no way to verify his story.

After listening to the prisoner tell his story it is the interrogator's call as to when to show him the photographs.

During the presentation by the instructor I could readily see my advantage in the first few critical moments of the interrogation. Not having written anything down or consulted a map, I could casually announce a coffee break. Once I was out the door I could quickly walk the few steps to the Photography Room and consult my aerial photographs. I could then return to the interrogation room.

The interrogator can tell a lot from that initial interview, explained the instructor. When questioning the prisoner about the route from his country of origin to the point he was captured, we should first expect one of two responses, as follows.

Complete cooperation, supported by the prisoner's truthfulness in giving you his home-base-to-capture route, might indicate the prisoner's belief that if he cooperated fully with his captors he might be treated well, or at least escape being executed as a spy.

On the other hand lying and giving evasive and misleading answers to his route-of-entry questions usually indicated disdain for the interrogator and continued resistance by the prisoner.

Although these initial responses of captured espionage agents are couched in terms of generalizations, I did find upon my arrival at the 502 that by a three-to-one margin the captured North Korean agents and their minders tended to cooperate with us.

In the following chapter I will explain in some detail the reasons for this unexpected cooperation.

The Chalky White Liquid

On April 10, 1962, my first day as the new feature writer for the *Stars & Stripes*, I walked around the corner with my fellow reporters to have supper at the 502 mess hall.

Jon Powell, the feature writer whom I had been "hired" to replace, introduced me to some of the 502's prisoner interrogators while sotto voce cautioning me not to ever ask them about their jobs – or the reason each of them carried around a not exactly small bottle filled with a thick chalky white liquid.

In point of fact stated Jon Powell, once supper ended and we reporters were walking back to the newspaper office and thus out of hearing range of anyone in the 502, those bottles were the best way to distinguish between the prisoner interrogators and the support personnel of the 502. Whereupon Jon answered my silent Why? Inquiry in a manner that whetted my newspaper reporter's keen interest.

"There aren't more than six or seven prisoner interrogators at the 502," he explained. "It must be the most stressful job in Korea, and within six months or so after one arrives, he is being treated for ulcers. The white liquid is taken to calm the stomache."

Powell went on to tell me that as soon as the interrogation session ended at 4:00 p.m., the interrogators walked over to the mess hall for a large glass of cold milk, whose purpose was to once again calm the wall of the complaining stomache.

At that moment our discussion of the purpose of the generic form of Kaopectate and cold milk and their relationship to the stresses resulting from the daily demands of interrogating enemy agents was indeed academic, because my serious interest in prisoner interrogation remained dormant until about six months into my tour of duty with the *Stars & Stripes*.

Chapter 13

◇◇◇◇◇

First Interrogation

At around noon on the day of my arrival at Kimpo Airport, the interrogator who had met me inside the terminal and I arrived at the main gate of the 502. The interrogator introduced me to the two M.P.s manning the gate, as the "new man," and we were waved through.

"Let's find you a bunk and drop off your duffel bag," said the interrogator. "Then we'll stop in at headquarters and you can meet with the colonel.

On the way from the airport, and before I could start asking my six dozen questions of curiosity, my driver had cautioned me against asking questions about the operation of the 502, stating that most of my questions were those that should be addressed to the commander of the 502.

Inside one of the Quonset huts we found a bunk and a locker for my valuables.

"At the moment there are seven interrogators, including you. You're gonna be kidded about this for sure, but even though you told me you just turned twenty-five, you don't look a day over twenty."

"It seems to have always been a problem, this endless youth thing," I said. "For fifteen months before joining army intelligence, I was the feature writer for the *Stars & Stripes*, and the high-ranking officers including generals whom I had to interview asked me whether I was the reporter's *Jeep driver*. And they were serious. It happened so often that I got used to it. It's not a problem."

"Well regardless of your age, if you weren't good at what you do you certainly wouldn't be here. It's a huge responsibility."

It suddenly came to me that his last comment, about interrogating communist spies being "a huge responsibility," might well prove to have a ring of truth to it. I wondered.

And this aspect of the job, this great "responsibility," was the very first thing the colonel stressed to me at our initial meeting early on the afternoon of my arrival at the 502.

"Provost, always remember that these are North Korean *spies* you are interrogating, not soldiers. When you initially meet one who has been recently captured, the clothes he is wearing are the ones he was wearing at the time the Korean army apprehended him. And historically-speaking, what is the fate of a captured spy?"

"The teaching staff at Ft. Holabird went over this with us, colonel. In South Korea the fate of any North Korean spy is execution," I said. It was at this very moment that the full meaning of my mission leapt up and hit me smack-dab in the face. I felt myself leaving the theoretical world behind. This was serious business.

Suddenly my year studying Korean at the Defense Language Institute and my 8-week course in prisoner interrogation at the U.S. Army Intelligence Center in Baltimore became quite academic, and these experiences seemed to fade away and become what they all along were intended to be, i.e., preparation for the *reality* I would face beginning the morning following the day of my arrival at the 502. Be careful what you wish for...

Layout of the 502

Upon my arrival at the 502 following completion of the 8-week course at Ft. Holabird, Maryland I learned that the prisoners were led from their Quonset huts at the corner of the compound, across the yard to the Interrogation Center (I.C.) at 8:00 a.m., five days per week.

The morning interrogation session ended promptly at 12:00 noon. The prisoners were led one at a time back to their Quonset huts, and lunch was delivered to them by the South Korean Army guards. The afternoon interrogation session began at 1:00 p.m. and ended at 4:00 p.m., five days per week.

The mess hall and the 502 headquarters offices were located in the same large one-story building, that was situated to the left as one entered the compound via the main gate.

The prisoners were housed in small Quonset huts located on the far side of the compound, one prisoner to a hut in order to prevent any communication among them. The distance between the headquarters-mess hall building and the nest of Quonset huts housing the prisoners was great enough that a person with excellent eyesight standing in front of the mess hall could not identify a person standing in front of one of the Quonset huts.

The Interrogation Center (I.C.) was situated roughly midway but somewhat off-center of a straight line connecting the three buildings in question. Our barracks, that actually were also Quonset huts, were located about fifty yards from the I.C., and the showers and toilet facilities were on a lower level but adjacent to the barracks. The interior of all these Quonset huts was heated by "space heaters" using oil.

The Interrogation Center was housed in a building standing alone, not inside a Quonset hut. A hallway divided the interior into two sides. We referred to the rooms in which we performed the interrogations as interrogation "rooms." However a more apt description would have been interrogation "booths."

At the rear of the interrogation rooms was situated the Photography Room where the U2 aerial photographs were laid out on long tables, with large magnifiers resting above them.

Deciding on A Method of Interrogation

As we were taught in Baltimore, each prisoner interrogator must settle on the method of interrogation which he finds more effective. This is the same decision a police detective in civilian life must make when interrogating suspects in a criminal case. Good cop – bad cop and all that follows.

So does the interrogator threaten and cajole a North Korean espionage agent from the very beginning of the interview?

Or does he adopt a conciliatory approach, letting the prisoner know that the interrogator understands and empathizes with the unfortunate man's plight?

As mentioned earlier, regardless of his background every interrogator in army intelligence, prior to being posted to Company A, 502 Military

Intelligence Battalion, had to attend the 8-week prisoner interrogation course at Ft. Holabird.

Eight weeks of play-acting in Baltimore is ample time for the student to experiment first-hand with the different approaches to interrogation and settle on the one with which he feels more comfortable.

At the 502 each American interrogator was paired with a Korean intelligence officer of at least the rank of colonel, and who spoke unaccented English fluently. These pairings were on a permanent basis and the Korean Army colonel I met the morning following my arrival, 47-year-old Colonel Kim, proved to be a very capable interrogator. We worked as a team throughout my sixteen-month tour at the 502, from early August 1964 to early November 1965.

My method of prisoner interrogation had been established long before I even began the 8-week course at Ft. Holabird in Baltimore.

My dad died on February 6, 1946. My mother could not properly care for seven children, so six months after his death, in August 1946 my older sister, age 9, was sent to live at historic Oxford Orphanage. I followed six months later, on February 15, 1947, at age seven, and several years later my younger brother Pete came along.

Oxford Orphanage was – and to this day still is – owned and operated by the Masonic Order of North Carolina. There was a cap on the number of students at 346.

In 2005 I wrote and published the only definitive history describing life at Oxford during the decade February 15, 1947 – February 15, 1957. It was an instant best-seller, was entitled *Reflections in an Orphan's Eye*, and subtitled *A Decade at Oxford 1947-1957*.

The memoir is 620 pages long, and among other things chronicles the verbal and physical abuses suffered by other children and myself at the hands of oftentimes uneducated, vindictive and abusive cottage counselors, work supervisors and teachers.

Because even at an early age I keenly observed the mistreatment of very young, disadvantaged children at the hands of uncaring adults, I was able to pick up on the defiant responses of many of these children.

The resentment to verbal mistreatment on the part of the children was quite palpable, and many of these youngsters developed personality traits that could best be described by a team of child psychiatrists completing a doctorate in Aberrant Behavior.

Therefore at the time of my arrival at Ft. Holabird I already knew the method of interrogation I would employ with captured North Korean espionage agents. My task was to extract information from the prisoner pertaining to his mission, his contacts in South Korea and the route he had followed on the way to his point of capture.

I knew of several ways to best obtain this crucial information. I decided to treat with respect an enemy I had never seen before and whose mission to kill South Koreans and American soldiers had been interrupted only by the vigilance of the South Korean Army.

"Colonel Kim has held off beginning to interrogate this next prisoner for two days, knowing you were on your way to Seoul," explained the colonel. "Let's walk over to the Interrogation Center. You can meet Col. Kim, then we'll have the new prisoner brought over."

Ten minutes later the colonel, Col. Kim of the ROK Army CID and I were seated at a small table inside an interrogation room. The colonel made the introductions, then turned to me.

"If there are no questions, then I'll leave and have the guards bring over the prisoner," he said.

"I'm ready sir," I said. "Anything I need, I'll ask Col. Kim here." I motioned to Col. Kim with a nod of my head and he returned a nod of agreement and understanding. The colonel departed, leaving Col. Kim and I facing one another across the narrow table.

"Col. Kim, do you usually shake hands with a prisoner the first time you meet him?"

"No I don't. But that's up to you," said the colonel. "I see nothing wrong with this gesture."

"Are you a coffee-drinker?" I asked.

"Yes, we Koreans of course prefer tea. However since nearly all Americans drink coffee, and a lot of it, I've grown to like it."

"Are you referring to the *coffee* or to the *sugar*?"

This comment provoked an instant and embarrassed laugh on the colonel's part. "Why I suppose the sugar," he said, this being the only answer he could honestly give. So within a few minutes I explained my idea

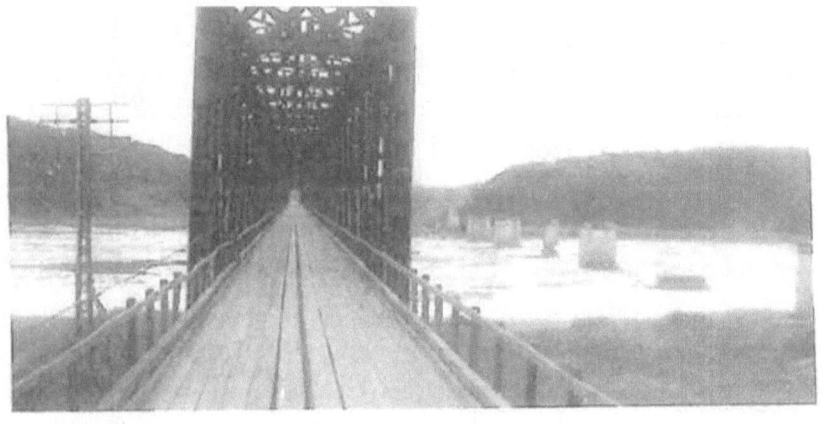

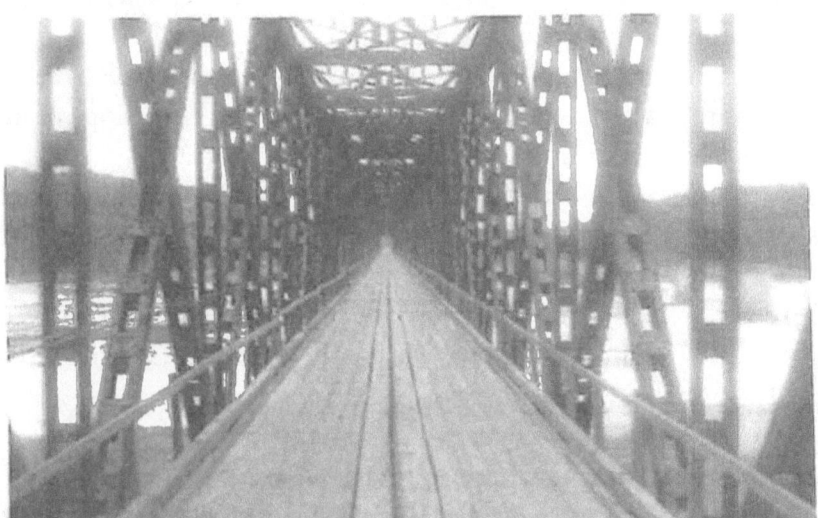

Bridge of No Return spanning a raging river just south of the DMZ (Demilitarized Zone) in First Cavalry Division country, Winter 1962. Note the.stone supports to the right that had carried a bridge during pre-Korean War times. Note the heavy wooden planks that had been placed over the railroad tracks in converting the metal trestle into a vehicle bridge.

The width of the river can be appreciated by noting how far away is the vanishing point of the trestle.

My Reasoning Re Coffee

In the early 1960s South Korea was still a very poor country. Because very little sugar cane was produced, the sources of the products used to produce sugar were almost nonexistent, mainly from beets.

If an American or other Westerner ordered coffee at a restaurant or tea house, the waitress would bring the cup of coffee and bowl of sugar on a tray, then depart, certain that the customer would take just a spoonful of sugar and no more.

If a Korean entered the same restaurant or tea house and ordered coffee, the waitress would bring the cup of coffee and bowl of sugar. She would place the cup of coffee on the table, then measure *only one* teaspoon of sugar. She would put the sugar into the coffee, stir the coffee and sugar, then walk away, wisely taking the bowl of sugar with her while leaving the unfortunate Korean salivating.

In Korea each American soldier was given a small ration book monthly. The ration book did not pay for the item, but allowed the G.I. to purchase the item in the PX. One of these items was a two-pound bag of sugar.

Because in most cases the soldier really did not need the sugar, he could (and usually did) sell the bag of sugar for between $20 and $30 to any restaurant or tea house throughout the country.

Recall that during this same period (early 1960s) communist North Korea was likely much poorer even than South Korea, so these captured espionage agents were likely the most sugar-starved people in all of Southeast Asia. I fully intended to use this fact to my advantage, beginning that very afternoon. Either my ambitious plan would work, or it wouldn't. But it was worth a try.

The fate of every communist espionage agent captured in South Korea was known throughout both North Korea and South Korea. These North Koreans were wearing *civilian* clothes, not North Korean Army uniforms. Thus they were spies, and their penalty was execution, usually by firing squad.

After more than half a century it is still difficult to put into words the thoughts that passed through my mind the afternoon the South Korean Army M.P.s opened the door to the interrogation room and ushered the frightened prisoner inside. They seated him across from us, then quietly departed.

Col. Kim opened his notebook and jotted down a few meaningless items. The 28-year-old prisoner watched the notebook, which didn't do him any good because the colonel was writing in English.

Addressing the prisoner by the name he had given the ROK Army soldiers who had captured him late the previous day, I extended my right hand across the table and spoke in crisp Korean:

"I am Officer Smith. I'm pleased to meet you."

He shook hands, his grip having the firmness of a wet dishrag and just as soggy, both indicating a high degree of apprehension.

"Before we get started, would you like a cup of coffee with sugar?" I asked politely. He answered in the affirmative. I arose and rapped on the door to the booth. When the Korean M.P. opened the door I asked him for three cups of coffee with sugar.

In that era, at every table in every mess hall on every military post in the U.S. stood an eight-inch high glass cylinder filled with pure cane sugar. Moments later the door opened and the M.P. entered. He placed the tray on the table between us. It contained three steaming mugs of coffee, three spoons and the glass cylinder of sugar.

Sugar was dispensed via a hole in the top of the cylinder, that was made of silver metal. Col. Kim poured about a teaspoonful of the sugar into his mug, stirred it briskly, then took a large swallow. I followed suit, then looked across at the prisoner. Ever since the M.P. entered the booth and placed the tray on the table, the sugar-deprived, mesmerized espionage agent had not been able to tear his gaze from that sugar dispenser.

"Go ahead," I encouraged, moving the sugar dispenser closer to him. He picked up the dispenser and poured in about twice the amount Col. Kim and I had taken.

After pouring this into his coffee and stirring the mixture it suddenly came to the prisoner that he had dissolved the sugar in his coffee, and the sudden disappointment on his face was palpable. He didn't want the coffee; all he wanted was the "fix" the large amount of refined cane sugar would give him.

Suddenly I had him just where I wanted him to be: I became his best friend.

"Go right ahead," I encouraged as I slid the sugar cylinder across the table toward him. "Take as much as you like." (*ma-um dae-ro*). And to my relief he did.

He upended the cylinder, and before he reluctantly ceased pouring I could see a mound of white sugar appearing at the top of the coffee.

Up to this point Col. Kim, according to our plan, had neither looked directly at the prisoner nor had he spoken to him. I asked Col. Kim if he would carry the tray and *two* coffee mugs to the back room. He agreed and left the room closing the door behind him, while the prisoner maintained a death-grip on the handle of his coffee mug full of sugar.

Strict rules of the interrogation center mandated that *both* interrogators, in this case Col. Kim and I, must be present during the interrogation session.

However Col. Kim did not carry the tray to the room down the hall. According to our plan he gave the tray to one of the M.P.s, then observed and listened to the conversation through the two-way mirror. He heard the following, both sides of the conversation in Korean.

"When you left your training base in North Korea, did your superiors inform you of your fate should you be captured?"

"Yes, they said I would be shot as a spy."

"Did they tell you to kill yourself rather than be captured?"

"Yes they did."

"Then why didn't you kill yourself?"

"Because I wanted to live."

"Well you still don't have to be shot as a spy."

"How is this? What do you mean?"

"The Korean officer who just stepped out is the supervisor of all the interrogators. He and I are close friends. If you decide to cooperate fully, I'll convince him to recommend a 20-year prison term rather than execution. They always follow his recommendation. You think about it and let me know. But don't let my friend know that you and I have discussed anything."

Minutes later Col. Kim returned. He sat at the table and the interrogation began. There were a number of ways to determine whether the prisoner was "cooperating fully." We would know.

Wonsan, North Korea

In the 1960s Wonsan, North Korea was important for a number of reasons. It was one of the largest seaports on the east coast, and boasted a fairly deep harbor. The North Korean Army and the North Korean Navy both maintained fortified bases in the area.

And most important of all, at one time or other every North Korean espionage agent had spent time in Wonsan, and most espionage missions into South Korea were launched from this port city though not necessarily directly from there.

Because of this situation, with the assistance of accurate and timely U2 aerial photographs the 502 interrogators knew Wonsan and the surrounding area as well as they knew any part of North Korea. And with cumulative intelligence gleaned from captured espionage agents we knew of the existence and mission of all North Korean military units in the area surrounding Wonsan.

In great detail.

Just as important to the intelligence analysts, these espionage agents, in order to get to Wonsan and from there to launch an operation into South Korea, must have been coming *from somewhere*.

Once we had established this beginning point, this "somewhere" as it were, we could call for aerial photographs to be taken at successive intervals on that town or area in order to track the activity and from this hopefully learn the mission of military units in that area. Thus the rule:

In order to get *to* a place, a person must have been coming *from* another place. Why?

The answer to this critical question came from previously-captured espionage agents. Although these espionage teams (at first comprised of the espionage *agent* and his two *minders*) set out from Wonsan, they trained for the mission at other, more secret bases in North Korea.

As one might suspect, the North Koreans had their own counterespionage teams in Wonsan, lying in wait for the appearance of any unfamiliar faces roaming the back alleys of this major port town.

Thus at the beginning of the interrogation the prisoner was faced with a decision. He could start lying, but if his deceit were exposed likely there would go any chance of escaping his fate – being executed as a spy.

However if he cooperated he might (he believed) spend the next twenty years in a South Korean prison. But he would be alive. And somewhere in his decision I couldn't help but think that the coffee mug full of sugar had helped him make up his mind. Finally he looked up at Col. Kim and me.

"I have decided to answer your questions," he said. *Touche'*.

The Three-man Teams

During the 1960s communist spies infiltrating South Korea via the steep and often treacherous East Sea coastline quite often came ashore as a three-man team, comprised of an espionage *agent* and his two *minders*. This method had begun to change by the time I left Korea in November 1965. More on this later.

Only the espionage *agent* knew the details of the mission. He was always *unarmed*.

The two minders knew only what they had been told by the espionage agent. They took their orders from the agent, except that the three always stayed together. They never split up. Not for any reason. In theory anyway.

In the event a ROK (Republic of Korea) Army patrol spotted the trio and a gunfight ensued, the two minders were under orders to execute the agent to prevent his being captured, then to commit suicide to avoid their own capture. Col. Kim took over the interrogation of the prisoner.

"How did you get to South Korea?"

"We went aboard a fishing boat north of Wonsan. The boat went far out to sea, then turned south. We were so far out we could not see land."

"How did you get to shore?"

"We were put onto a large rubber raft at night. We could see the lights on shore from the South Korean village of Sokcho. The two men with me used the paddles and we headed for shore. We were supposed to let the air out of the rubber raft before we reached shore, and sink the raft."

"Where are the two men who came with you?"

"One of the men was armed, just like me. The other man carried the money, and this man was not armed," he said.

"I was afraid the man with the gun would shoot me. In the darkness I grabbed the large knife from him and stabbed both of them to death."

We had us a *minder*, not an *agent*, because an agent would not have been armed.

As Col. Kim explained to me after the prisoner had been returned to his Quonset hut at 4:00 p.m., it had become standard practice for the trio of spies to carry with them large amounts of Korean and American money, usually $30,000 in hundreds and another $30,000 in Korean paper money called the *won*. These large amounts of cash were earmarked for delivery to North Korean agents in hiding in South Korea. During the 1960s the South Korean *won* was fairly stable on the world financial market. However American currency ruled world finance and to your average Korean, American dollars were literally "as good as gold."

A student can learn a lot in eight weeks if he is motivated and is taught by dedicated instructors. At Ft. Holabird both these situations existed, plus I had a leg up on most of the American prisoner interrogators at the 502.

These definite advantages included the fact that I was one of only two interrogators who had been stationed in South Korea prior to attending the Defense Language Institute for a year and the eight-week prisoner interrogation course at Ft. Holabird.

Filing the Daily Interrogation Summary

Thus when I walked into class the first morning at the Defense Language Institute I already spoke passable Korean, knew the *lay of the land* so to speak and was already familiar with the customs and daily lives of Koreans in general.

At the end of that first day inside the interrogation center and after the prisoner had been returned to his Quonset hut for the night, a smiling Col. Kim shook hands with me.

"I must admit, Specialist Provost, that I never would have thought of the sugar-in-the-coffee trick. But I think it will work."

"Well I hope so," I said. "Now what do we do with the rest of the day?"

"Let's sit here at the table and discuss what I will send to the South Korean Army and you'll "twix" (teletype) to G-2 at the Pentagon in Washington, D.C."

It took about fifteen minutes of discussion of our abbreviated interrogation session before we had it ready for me to type my summary.

"I can tell from your writing that you get to the point quickly," remarked the colonel.

"I have an advantage here," I answered. "Before I joined U.S. Army Intelligence I was the feature writer for the *Stars & Stripes* for fifteen months. I was writing my articles just about every day and I learned to be precise and get to the point."

"It seems to me that questioning people for your newspaper articles is a lot like interrogating an espionage agent," said the colonel.

"I believe so," I said. "In both cases we are out to get information. The biggest difference is that the person being questioned for the newspaper article wants to *give* you information whereas the communist agent wants to *keep* this information from you."

"We'll type our summary for the day over at headquarters," said the colonel. "Let's walk over now if you are finished."

"I wouldn't change anything," I said. "By the way, who approves the interrogation summary before I type it?"

"No one approves it. You have been well-trained as an interrogator, so nobody can order you to change anything in your summary. What is written is just what the prisoner told you. This is the reason you and I discuss the case before you type it, to make certain my conclusions are as close to yours as is possible."

I walked into headquarters where I observed several interrogators seated at small desks busily typing their summaries for the day. I sat and prepared to type.

"Make sure you have enough carbon paper," advised one of the interrogators. "You need to keep two copies. The original goes to the Twix Center when we have gathered them all together." I inserted three clean sheets of typing paper and two sheets of carbon paper into the manual typewriter and began typing my summary.

After fifteen months of writing my stories at the *Stars & Stripes* almost on a daily basis I had become quite an efficient typist. In fifteen minutes I had typed – single-spaced of course – my *Interrogation Summary*, that included my analysis of what the facts showed and whether I believed the prisoner was being truthful with his answers.

Sitting at the narrow desk hunched over the typewriter, I recalled the very capable instructors at Ft. Holabird and the importance of giving my first-hand opinion as to the veracity of the prisoner.

"You are the person who has just finished interrogating the enemy. Thus you must have an opinion as to whether we should believe any of what he told you. This opinion is very important to the military analysts who weren't present at the interrogation," said the instructor.

The Twix Center at Yongsan

As noted above, interrogations came to an abrupt halt at 4:00 p.m. sharp. After conforming our summary of the day's interrogation, Col. Kim departed to deliver his Daily Summary to the ROK (Republic of Korea) Army's Intelligence Analysts in Seoul, and I walked to headquarters to prepare my typed Daily Summary for delivery to the U.S. Eighth Army's large "twix" (teletype) center, located on the Yongsan compound in downtown Seoul.

The Daily Summaries of the interrogators were time-sensitive, in that the briefcase carrying them had to arrive at the Twix Center before 6:00 p.m.

Each interrogator was responsible for typing his own Daily Summary, then signing the document. I was one of the fastest typists, having typed all my dozens of articles I wrote as a feature writer for the *Stars & Stripes* for fifteen months, so I was eager to assist the slower typists with their Summaries.

For two reasons. First the interrogators were friends, and they appreciated the help. Second, it gave me an opportunity to see the other interrogators' work, because every North Korean espionage agent had his own story to tell.

Once all the Daily Summaries had been typed, signed and ready to go, they were placed inside a briefcase. The briefcase was locked and two M.P.s (one driving, the other riding shotgun) and one of the interrogators (sitting in the back seat of the Jeep) drove from the 502 north across the long Han River Bridge to the Twix Center at U.S. Eighth Army headquarters in Yongsan.

With the interrogator carrying the locked briefcase, he and the two M.P.s entered the front door of the large Twix Center and approached the long counter.

The reason the interrogator carried the briefcase was that the prisoner interrogator possessed Top Secret Security Clearance whereas the M.P.s held only Secret Security Clearances.

The "Twix Center" is short for "Teletype Center." The interrogator and the two M.P.s had to remain in the reception center while the clerk signed in and sent the teletype across the ocean to G-2 Headquarters in the Pentagon. Once this had been accomplished the clerk returned the documents to the briefcase and handed the briefcase to the interrogator for the return trip to the 502.

Timing was all-important to what we interrogators were trying to accomplish. Our notes and Daily Summaries were received at the Pentagon, where they were scoured by analysts. If an analyst required more specific information or needed clarification on a specific point, he would type out his needs, then prepare updated requests and comments. Once these reports had been collected, they were twixed back over the airwaves to the Twix Center at Yongsan from the Pentagon.

Prior to the beginning of interrogation the following morning at 8:00, the interrogator checked the prisoner's G-2 folder, then formulated the questions they needed for us to ask the prisoner.

Not all the messages from the intelligence analysts at G-2 were in the form of questions. Often they were suggestions as to following a certain line of questioning. After all, the interrogators were the eyes and ears of the intelligence analysts, and the latters' requests and suggestions took precedence over our daily interrogations.

If a request from G-2 was marked *Urgent*, we had to question the prisoner as soon as the interrogation session began at 8:00 a.m. The follow-up Report was typed (again by the interrogator) and the M.P.s and the interrogator were off to Yongsan to twix the "Urgent" report to G-2.

Thus every day was a Pressure Day at the 502, and it was nigh onto impossible to do our job well without succumbing to the stress.

Could *burnout* be far behind? And to think I had only gotten started!

Spooks *and Their Role at the 502*

Perceptive chap that I was I realized shortly after I had arrived at the 502 and met them, that the two polite and modest "suits" were from the CIA.

Each of the men could speed-read a 6-page Interrogation Summary in ten seconds flat, even pointing out several spelling or punctuation errors along the way. Intelligence as a major component of a person's persona always impressed me. Still does.

If either of the two ever engaged in any cloak-and-dagger shenanigans (spy stuff), you certainly couldn't prove it by me. And you could see the dedication in their eyes, that never left my face until they said, "Thanks Provost, we'll be in touch."

When I arrived at the 502 compound upon my return to Korea following my tours of duty at the Defense Language Institute and the U.S. Army Intelligence Center in Baltimore, I received the same introduction as did any new interrogator.

"I will assume that you might wonder who are the two civilians you'll see visiting the Interrogation Center, Provost. We'll let you guess as to where they are from, but you may share any of your interrogation notes with them. They are the reason we type our Interrogation Summaries in triplicate."

Thus following sixteen months of interacting with these two, every prisoner interrogator knew without asking, just who were these two CIA agents and what was their mission.

Chapter 14

◇◇◇◇◇

End of First Day at the 502

At the end of my first day at the 502 one of the officers, a captain, met me inside my interrogation room.

"Provost, you should be the ideal interrogator," he began. "Your ROK Army counterpart, Col. Kim, is quite impressed with your knowledge of the Korean language and the fact that you have a detailed road map of both North Korea and South Korea stored inside your head."

"Thank you sir," I replied.

At this point I believe I expected to receive some sort of indoctrination into my new job, together with the details of the results I was expected to achieve. I recalled having received such a welcome at both the Defense Language Institute and at the beginning of the eight-week Prisoner Interrogation Course at Ft. Holabird. An *overview*, they called it.

Such an expected introduction not having been made I decided to give the captain a little verbal nudge to get him back on track. Welcome to reality, Provost.

"Who is going to give me the details of the operation of the interrogation center?" I inquired. "First of all, who is my immediate supervisor who will be reviewing my reports?"

At this point I sensed an almost imperceptible pause in our conversation. Not knowing exactly how to end this impasse I elected to say nothing. I waited. Finally he seemed to understand my question.

"As far as the operation of the I.C. (Interrogation Center) is concerned, someone will go over this with you after breakfast tomorrow morning," said the captain.

"However as to your second question, the answer is that you do not have an immediate supervisor in the generally accepted sense of the word, and no one is going to review your Interrogation Summaries in the sense one might understand the meaning of *review*. So this is the way we operate."

At this point allow me to paraphrase what the captain had to say.

First of all, who would be available to review and pass on my work anyway?

Nobody. Because the interrogation of foreign agents is such a personal undertaking. I had been taught my skill by expert interrogators, and I could speak Korean, if not fluently, at least I felt confident that I could communicate with these communists. Therefore if an American army officer attempted to critique my work, he wouldn't know where to begin. I was the expert and the officer was not. Rank did not determine expertise in the field of prisoner interrogation any more than it determined who should be granted a Top Secret Security Clearance.

The reasons I had spent a year at the Defense Language Institute studying Korean six hours a day, five days a week, plus two hours of homework each night, then eight weeks of instruction in prisoner interrogation techniques, was in order for me to *hit the ground running* the day I arrived at the 502.

Once the captain explained it to me this way everything made sense. Plainly stated the sole purpose of forty or so 502 troops was to support a half dozen prisoner interrogators in the furtherance of the latters' mission.

"There is one thing of which we remind every new prisoner interrogator just in case he missed out on this during his course of instruction at Ft. Holabird," said the captain.

Whereupon he repeated the U.S. Army's proscription against the mistreatment of captured North Korean espionage agents.

"You can threaten the espionage agent as much as you like," said the captain. "You just cannot strike him, not with a weapon and not with your hand."

Allowing his comment to register for a moment or so, he continued.

"Each interrogator develops his own techniques. I of course am not a prisoner interrogator, but as I walk along the narrow hallways of the I.C., I can tell that the interrogators are using different methods. *Whatever works* is my motto. From this point forward, you're on your own."

"I became a prisoner interrogator because I believed I would be good at what I do," I said. "But believe me captain, I would not be sitting here now if I were expected to use physical force to get the information I need."

"The question naturally arises however, what do we do when the North Korean espionage *agent*, or one of his two *minders*, refuses to give us information that we know he has or should have," he added rhetorically.

"Once you and your interrogation partner Col. Kim agree that the prisoner refuses to answer your questions, Col. Kim will notify his superiors in the ROK (Republic of Korea) Army. That same night three Korean Army M.P.s will arrive in a paddy wagon. They will collect the prisoner, and return him at daybreak the following morning."

"Do you ever learn what happened to the prisoner?" I asked with morbid curiosity.

"I'm glad you asked that question," responded the captain. "The answer is that we never ask the prisoner or your counterpart Col. Kim. We treat it for what it is – an internal Korean problem with an internal Korean solution."

"That's all I need to know," I said. "Mum's the word."

The Final Interrogation Summary

A lost minder was as likely to be apprehended by a policeman in a small town as by a South Korean soldier on patrol. In my travels throughout the country during my 15-month tour of duty with the *Stars & Stripes*, I observed that even in small towns there were at least two policemen. And these policemen were constantly on the lookout for any new faces in town.

Once we determined that the minder could add little to the interrogation – "we" being Col. Kim and myself – I reported to the officers that I would be writing the *Final Interrogation Summary* within days.

The reason for this notification was to allow the staff to tentatively schedule our interrogation team – Col. Kim and I – another prisoner. This was often easier said than done. However during the early and mid 1960s there were never more than six or seven interrogators posted to Company A, 502 Military Intelligence Battalion. Certainly kept us busy anyway.

Even without asking however, about a month after I began interrogating prisoners, I had just finished breakfast one morning and was walking across the grassy lawn from the mess hall to the I.C., when in my peripheral vision I noticed a prisoner being escorted from his Quonset hut cell to the I.C. for the morning interrogation session.

The prisoner was literally hopping on one foot, then the other, as quickly and as gingerly as possible, and I could readily see the expression of pain and anguish on his face. Two weeks later the prisoner was still hopping. And he was telling the American interrogator anything the interrogator wanted to hear.

You Do It Your Way, Sir.

As mentioned earlier all branches of the military and different units within the branches were represented at both the Defense Language Institute and the Prisoner Interrogation Course at the Army Intelligence Center in Baltimore.

In 1964 the Vietnam War was in full bloom, and many of the U.S. Army Special Forces soldiers who we met while we were studying Korean and they Vietnamese at the Defense Language Institute, were in our class at Ft. Holabird because, as noted above the Prisoner Interrogation Course was not geared to any specific language.

The officer instructors at Ft. Holabird really knew their subject, and they crammed a lot of reason and knowledge into the 8-week course on Prisoner Interrogation Theory and Practice.

The techniques of sleep deprivation and threats of physical harm were discussed for the sake of inclusiveness; however every instructor who touched on these techniques questioned their effectiveness and urged the students to do likewise. I recall one morning when the instructor had just begun a lecture on the futility of torture during interrogations.

At this point one of the half dozen Special Forces soldiers raised his hand, and the instructor acknowledged him.

"We in the Special Forces fully understand where you're coming from Sir, but often we cannot follow these precautions as most of our work demands information immediately, such as the location of their Viet Cong troops and the number of weapons they possess. So respectfully sir, you do it your way and we in the Special Forces will do it ours." Enough said.

The Substitute Interrogators

As noted earlier I was the only graduate of the 47-week language course at Monterey, California and the prisoner interrogation course in Baltimore, Maryland, who had been posted to the 502. Because, as they informed me, all the 502 needed at the time was one more prisoner interrogator.

Two months after my arrival at the 502, I was still adjusting to my new duties and realizing quickly the reason the prisoner interrogators walked around the base carrying an eight-ounce bottle filled with that chalky-white liquid and stopped by the mess hall every mid-afternoon for a tall glass of cold milk.

At noon each day during the week the interrogators broke for lunch. As we washed our hands and walked the short distance to the mess hall, the Korean guards marched the prisoners one at a time back to their Quonset huts, where they ate lunch delivered by the guards.

Anyway on this particular day, as I entered the mess hall I heard a familiar voice call out to me in passable Korean:

"Pak Il Byung, kidadi-seyo. Oregan man-e." (Corporal Park, please wait. It's been a long time.)

I turned to see two of the men who had been with me at both the language school and the prisoner interrogation course. I shook hands with each of them and we walked into the mess hall.

"So you two will be interrogators?" I asked as we found seats at a table.

"No, I'm afraid we're not here as prisoner interrogators, or even Korean linguists," said one of the men.

"Care to explain?" I asked with what I'm certain was a puzzled expression on my face.

"The best way to describe it is to say we're the *backup* interrogators. We'll have jobs to do on post, and if you lose an interrogator you'll already have his replacement here."

"Now in addition to drawing his regular salary, the interrogator draws two proficiency-pay units," I said. "He receives one pro-pay unit for being a Korean linguist and an additional one for being a prisoner interrogator. Each pro-pay unit is $300. So each month he receives his regular pay plus an extra $600. Will you receive these pro-pays also?"

"Yes, they explained to us that we will receive these pro-pays, because this is determined by our M.O.S. (Military Occupational Skill), even though we are not presently doing this work."

"Well I'm glad to see you guys here, and if you need any help finding your way around just let me know," I said.

"Can we tell you a secret, Al? We wouldn't want it to become common knowledge around base, but neither of us ever really wanted to become prisoner interrogators, so if they never need to call on us, this would be just fine."

"Mum's the word," I said. "Your secret's safe with me."

The camaraderie among the three of us stemmed from the friendship we developed while attending the Defense Language Institute and the Prisoner Interrogation Course at Ft. Holabird. This feeling remained the anchor of our friendship throughout my tour of duty at the 502, and I treated them as equals in our life on the compound.

Chapter 15

◇◇◇◇◇

Interrogation Techniques

Three months into my new duties as a prisoner interrogator I was certain I knew the Secret of the Chalky White Liquid. As discussed earlier somehow I expected to take a course called "Introduction to Interrogating a Prisoner Whose First Language is Not English," or better still, "Interrogation of Communist Espionage Agents Made Simple." Or something along those lines anyway. But alas, this did not occur.

A more apt description of this third-world adventure was that it was like being thrown to the lions, straight out of *Ben-Hur*. Talk about *total immersion!*

When even today my memory conjures up images of my sixteen months at the 502, the one descriptive word that best signifies what we were subjected to was *Pressure. Daily*, and lots of it.

Our master was not the U.S. Army or the 502 or the commandant of the 502.

No, the reason for our existence was the Pentagon's demanding *G-2 Section*. And those analysts were the reason our interrogations ended at 4:00 p.m. sharp Monday through Friday.

As soon as the prisoner was marched back to his cell in his Quonset hut, Col. Kim and I conformed our data gathered that day. The English version and the Korean version had to say the same thing factually.

As soon as this was accomplished Col. Kim departed to make his report to South Korean Army Intelligence, and I carried my handwritten original to the headquarters building where I met the other interrogators and the two CIA agents. These CIA agents of course received a copy of everything we produced.

Along this chain of command that began with the interrogators and ended on the desk of a G-2 analyst, there was no *middle man*. In other words no one checked my interrogation notes nor my interpretation of the data, that was always required. I was expected to offer an on-site opinion based on first-hand knowledge gained through questioning an enemy agent seated no more than four feet across the table. It really boiled down in a nutshell to:

All things considered, did I believe what the enemy agent was telling me?

I was asked to err on the side of *caution*. There was no such thing as giving the enemy the benefit of the doubt.

Col. Kim early on stated that the North Korean agents trusted the Americans more than they did the Koreans. After discussing this fact Col. Kim and I thought of a way to use this to our advantage. If an enemy were lying, we could ask him literally the same question three times and come up with two different answers. As they were not intelligent, trained espionage agents none had ever received training in evasion tactics.

If during the interrogation we were uncertain of this agent's veracity, Col. Kim would tell me (in Korean) that he had to run a short errand and for me to suspend the interrogation until he returned. Col. Kim would close the door and walk down the hall, and the enemy agent and I could hear the colonel's footfalls on the wooden floor of the I.C.

Then the colonel would quietly return to the room and listen at the closed door as I, using my best conspirator's tone, would ask the agent whether there was anything he would like to tell me in the colonel's absence.

And just whom was the North Korean agent going to trust? On the first day of his interrogation I was the American soldier who had tacitly agreed to keep him supplied with refined white cane sugar. Thus any obligation the enemy agent believed he owed was to his benefactor, the kind American soldier who by the way never had even once raised his voice at the prisoner.

Col. Kim and I believed that if this ruse worked once – which it did – it would likely work again. And it did. And somewhere along the line I told Col. Kim the meaning of the American expression, *There's more than one way to skin a cat*.

It was all part of a game – admittedly a deadly one – of wits. If before Col. Kim's departure on his "short errand" down the hall, the prisoner had given us conflicting answers to our factual questions, in Col. Kim's absence I would draw the prisoner's attention to these discrepancies and then ask:

"I see that you have given two different answers to (such-and-such) question, I'm certain not on purpose. Now take your time and let me know which answer was your correct answer."

The Improbable Narrative – The Lie

The most difficult evasion tactic the prisoner could employ, according to the instructors at Ft. Holabird's Prisoner Interrogation Course, was to lie to the interrogator. For in order to tell a lie – regardless of how simple or complex – requires the prisoner to build a narrative, a false story that must now of necessity run parallel to the truthful one. And somehow the prisoner must convince the interrogator that *both* his narratives are true. And it simply cannot be done. *Prisoner Interrogation Techniques 101*.

One dead giveaway to a lying prisoner's deceit is to observe increasingly the interval of time between the interrogator's questions and the prisoner's responses. With each question asked, a liar's interval grows longer.

Col. Kim, who had been an interrogator for three years when I joined him in 1964, could determine after asking the prisoner five short questions whether he was being truthful. Yet rarely did the savvy colonel challenge the prisoner on this initial lie, opting to continue the interrogation, hoping to discover the *reason* for the prisoner to begin giving evasive, misleading answers.

We had to bear in mind two things pertinent to questioning both the better-educated espionage *agent* and the agent's less well-educated *minders*.

First we had to avoid the tendency – solely based on his education – to underestimate the agent or minder.

Aside from this however we always had to be mindful of the fact that the prisoner has been taught to mislead, as to both the facts and his intentions. The downside to this however is that when the prisoner starts lying, soon he cannot separate his lies from the truth.

Thus in confronting the prisoner with the two answers he has just given us, it is quite obvious that one of these answers cannot be the truth, leading to befuddlement on the prisoner's part. Except that now he is either apt to give a truthful answer, or else interject a third, different answer, a lie.

From this example it is quite understandable to see how difficult is the prisoner interrogator's job . Two words I never recall hearing during my 16-month stint at the 502 were "easy interrogation." They were all difficult. Quite.

During my 8-week course in Prisoner Interrogation and Aerial Photograph Analysis at Ft. Holabird, I had taken copious notes, that I reviewed prior to interrogating my first prisoner. Several points stood out almost as truisms, as follows:

One learns absolutely nothing while talking, but can learn almost everything while listening. Both the interrogator and the prisoner want the prisoner to speak freely, but for different reasons. The longer the prisoner talks the greater the chance he will slip up and provide damaging information. The prisoner's reason differs somewhat. Although he has been told by his officers in the North Korean Army that if captured he will be executed as a spy, the longer he talks the longer he lives – and hopes that by some miracle he might escape his fate.

There are some useful guidelines relating to making eye contact with a prisoner. If the prisoner avoids eye contact entirely, mark him down as a liar for certain, until he proves you wrong.

Initial eye contact, broken quickly by looking away, usually to the side of the dominant hand, indicates evasion. By making eye contact initially the prisoner is imploring the interrogator to believe him.

Constant, unwavering eye contact might indicate that the prisoner has been coached in deception tactics. In a normal conversation rarely will a prisoner employ constant, unwavering eye contact. It's quite unnatural.

However a prisoner who maintains eye contact with the interrogator *when responding to a direct question* may well be telling the truth.

Regardless of the above, the interrogator must be conscious of maintaining eye contact at all times. Failing to do this may lead to disastrous consequences.

A tactic used successfully by civilian trial attorneys I found to be effective in several situations at the 502. If you ask a prisoner a question and he answers the direct question, rather than ask another question, simply repeat one or two key words. Often the prisoner will make a question out of these words and will give pertinent answers thereto.

The instructors at the Ft. Holabird Army Intelligence Center had of course been correct. Prisoner of War interrogation is a learning process, and the first time you think you can approach the interrogation of Prisoner B in exactly the same manner as you just approached Prisoner A, you'll be in for a rude awakening. You are not dealing with a cookbook.

Furthermore the instructors cautioned, never assume that because of the different status of the prisoner and the interrogator, that you, the interrogator, necessarily control the course of the interrogation.

This proved to be true with my second prisoner, as we shall see.

Chapter 16

◇◇◇◇◇

Incompatible Goals of Agents and Minders

As soon as a captured North Korean spy was brought to the 502 it was essential to learn the status of the prisoner i.e., whether he was an *agent* or one of the agent's *minders*.

The success of the mission depended on the 3-man team remaining intact. Only one of the three, the agent, was privy to the details of the mission. And he in turn, was the only one of the trio who could find his way across country to the designated safehouse, nearly always the first stop on this perilous mission.

Information from numerous captured minders showed that in every case, the agent was the only one of the three who ever handled the money, that usually amounted to $30,000 in hundred-dollar bills and another $30,000 in Korean *won*.

Experience also indicated that what started out as a disciplined espionage mission fell apart at the moment of discovery by a ROK Army patrol. Because ninety percent of intelligence gathered on North Korea came from the 502 prisoner interrogations, South Korean patrols were ordered not to fire on suspected North Korean agents unless the enemy agents fired first.

The aspect of North Korean espionage that initially seemed out of kilter to me was when I discovered that the two minders were armed but the agent was not armed.

The agent understood that if the trio were discovered and the agent's capture appeared imminent, his two minders were under orders to first kill the agent in order to prevent his capture, then to commit suicide, because as they entered South Korea as spies in civilian clothes and not as soldiers in uniform, the penalty under South Korean law was death, nearly always by firing squad. There was no allowance under Korean law for extenuating circumstances, as we will see.

According to captured agents and minders, if the team were spotted by South Korean Army patrols the odds of them coming out of a firefight alive were nigh onto nonexistent. They would always be outnumbered because the South Korean Army patrols were reinforced patrols, operating on familiar ground. Thus the team's tactics when discovered centered on evasion and flight, not confrontation.

The problem communist espionage planners encountered was that the minder could not be trusted to end his own life. When threatened with capture, the agent would be more likely to kill his minders and surrender, in hopes that his life would be spared if he cooperated fully with the South Korean authorities. It was for these reasons that the agent was not armed but the minders were armed.

Indeed the first prisoner I interrogated, a minder, had killed his two comrades and then surrendered, hoping for more lenient treatment.

In Korea in the 1960s perhaps the most glaring misnomer was "a volunteer communist espionage agent." There simply was no such animal. One of the truisms circulating along the halls of the I.C. was that fifty percent of the captured North Korean spies initially resisted interrogation whereas we couldn't stop the other fifty percent from spilling their guts. The reason?

Among all the communist espionage agents held at the 502 during my sixteen months as an interrogator, and of which I was aware, not a single one admitted to having volunteered for the mission. And I came to believe them.

I compiled a few statistics in the I.C., and from these made some conclusions in this regard, empirically speaking of course.

One of the questions asked of each enemy agent was the extent of his education. I never met or heard of any *minder* who had ever attained the American equivalent of a high school education.

However the *agents* in the 3-man teams all appear to have completed the American equivalent of high school, and several came from the North Korean Army's officer ranks.

In addition the minders appeared to be an expendable breed. When quickly and thoroughly searched at the point of capture, none was found to be in possession of a road map, neither of North Korea nor South Korea.

Under questioning we discovered that upon becoming separated from the group the minder was "on his own," left to fend for himself, to be captured by the first policeman or army unit he encountered. Because the minder was not told anything concerning the details of the mission, he possessed no information affecting the mission one way or the other.

Expanding the Espionage Web

The communist three-man unit's primary goal upon making it safely ashore along the steep and heavily patrolled eastern coastline was to find its way to the safehouse, following the directions given to the *agent* just prior to leaving the port of Wonsan or other port.

The note to the agent contained written directions to the safehouse, usually located in a village or at the edge of a small town. The following account of the operation of a safehouse is based on interrogations of communist agents captured before they reached their destination.

The owner of the safehouse would report that an unknown Korean – believed to be a *South* Korean – rented the small house several weeks in advance of the 3-man espionage team's arrival in South Korea.

The renter then left the area and was never again seen by the owner of the house.

When the 3-man North Korean team arrived, the team entered, leaving the $30,000 in American money and the $30,000 in Korean *won* safely buried in the woods far away. Most of the large amount of money was being sent to communist agents already ensconced in safehouses throughout South Korea.

In the event the South Korean Army ;'patrols had spotted the North Koreans coming ashore in rubber rafts and rather than capture them, had decided to follow them to the safehouse, they would find nothing but an empty house.

If the South Korean Army patrols had not discovered and apprehended the 3-man espionage team, the renter of the house will have left enough food and water available for five days. If after five days no South Korean Army patrols had shown up at the safehouse, the communists would assume that the team had not been compromised, and they could safely resume the mission.

In the course of my tour of duty at the 502 I never was aware of the capture of a complete 3-man North Korean espionage team.

In addition my South Korean CIC (counterintelligence corps) counterpart Col. Kim could recall no enemy spy – either agent or minder – ever committing suicide. Apparently the will to live is cast in stone regardless of where one calls home.

However the act of killing one's team member, then surrendering to the South Korean Army patrols, appeared to be commonplace. We interrogators reasoned that this practice worked in the following manner.

Espionage mission planners back in Pyongyang, more likely through experience, never allowed any of the minders to handle the money. Upon arriving safely at the safe house in South Korea the minders were ordered to remain in the house while the agent located a hiding place for the money.

In addition it was nigh onto impossible for the two minders to collude in the murder of the agent, for two reasons. They had no money because the agent had hidden it. And the minders first met within ten days of the mission and were never left alone together. Thus there was never time enough for the two minders to establish a relationship of trust leading to collusion.

The minders realized they were the low men on the totem pole, that they were considered by their superiors back in North Korea to be expendable, i.e. excess baggage.

In addition they either believed before the mission began, or became convinced after the first shot fired that no way in Hades were they going to survive a firefight with a South Korean Army patrol.

Furthermore the minders would have a hard time killing the agent because once discovered, the agent took flight immediately. Thus the agent was fleeing from the South Korean Army patrol *and* from his own minders.

In this regard the minders routinely overestimated their own worth, simply because they could add very little of substance to what the agent knew.

Because the minder's mission was quite limited – executing the agent if his capture appeared imminent – he knew absolutely nothing of the mission, and if the trio were spotted and became separated upon landing by rubber raft on the coast, the minder would not even know how to make his way to the safehouse because only the agent possessed this information. Survival did not favor the expendable minder.

Chapter 17

◇◇◇◇◇

My First Prisoner's Execution

Col. Kim and I had interrogated our first prisoner daily for less than two months when we came to the inescapable conclusion that as a source of intelligence he had nothing further of value to add to his file.

The 28-year-old soldier possessed what we surmised was a sixth-grade education. He could add and subtract but even the rudiments of multiplication and division were foreign concepts. He had never traveled outside the province of his birth. Five years earlier the laborer had been drafted into the North Korean Army as a Private; at the time of his capture was still a Private, and most of his day had been spent performing manual labor.

All the relevant evidence pointed to the conclusion that the minder had only one purpose, which was to serve as an armed escort for the agent from the east coast to the safehouse, or else murder the agent if the trio were discovered en route. It was not worth the North Korean espionage planners' time and resources to hide the three men or to attempt to exfiltrate them by picking them up off the coast by means of a rubber raft. The two minders it appeared, had been "hung out to dry" by the mission planners back in Pyongyang.

The prisoner's only claim to fame had been his consistently high scores on the pistol and rifle range. The prisoner and we agreed that this was the reason he had been selected to train for two months as an espionage agent's minder.

The prisoner had not met his *fellow minder* and the espionage *agent* until ten days prior to the mission. His orders had been concise and to the point. He was to protect the agent. However if the trio was faced with capture he was to kill the agent and the other minder, then commit suicide.

And there were other subtle signs that our prisoner was a minder and not an agent. He had no maps of South Korea on his person and none were found discarded or hidden along his route from the coast. Furthermore the prisoner did not even know how to read a road map.

The only weapon he carried (in his trouser pocket) was a five-shot Chinese pistol, and he carried no reloads. The weapon had not been fired recently, according to the South Korean Army M.P.s. As with subsequent captured communist espionage agents, we interrogators were left with the impression they had been poorly trained and inadequately equipped for such a dangerous mission.

On the afternoon of the day the mission began the three men were driven to Wonsan, where they boarded a fishing trawler, whereupon he observed that the 4-man crew was armed with pistols. During the entire voyage the three were kept below deck, so he was unable to report on the route the boat followed to arrive on the eastern coast of South Korea under cover of darkness.

The South Korean Army patrols were under strict orders to refrain from attempting to question these espionage agents at the point of capture or on the way to the 502 compound.

Anytime a layman (non-interrogator) questioned a captured enemy agent the layman was giving the agent time to formulate questions he might be asked by an experienced interrogator once the prisoner arrived at the 502. These enemy agents and minders might have been somewhat lacking in intelligence but I don't believe I ever called one of them stupid. Again the fear of underestimating the enemy was on my mind constantly. *Caution* remained the name of the interrogator's game. I was the youngest interrogator; this fact kept me on my toes, and I always felt the need to prove myself.

Col. Kim and I interrogated my first prisoner for slightly less than two months. He had no reason to question the colonel's promise of a reprieve to avoid his execution, so he never again broached the subject. Nor did we.

As far as we knew the prisoner never intentionally misled us. He had no way of knowing that I had memorized a road map of both North Korea and South Korea. Yet in tracing his moves through North Korea including his place of birth and various landmarks, his map locations to and from these towns, roads and rivers conformed with what he told us.

Throughout his interrogation I was saddled with a recurring thought that he had not volunteered for this mission and he did not intend that any harm come to any American or South Korean. Or so he claimed.

Finally the time came to write and twix to G-2 my Final Interrogation Summary. Fleetingly I thought of giving the prisoner several Hershey chocolate bars I had purchased at the large PX (Post Exchange) at Eighth U.S. Army headquarters at Yongsan. However I deep-sixed that idea because he might be put on his guard that something was amiss.

Same with a parting handshake. The only time we shook hands had been when I greeted him at the first interrogation session. However such a gesture also would alert him to a change in routine.

Physical Abuse on the Road to Inchon

There were seven interrogators at the 502. From my first week on the compound I had heard rumors of "someone" assaulting the prisoners on the latters' last night on the base, and at other times.

And such a rumor, once having a basis and ample opportunity, eventually segued into more than rumor. The South Koreans' hatred of the North Koreans was a given, and for good reason – the North Koreans had entered South Korea for the purpose of murdering South Koreans and Americans and establishing espionage networks to do more of the same.

Thus the *basis* of these assaults was hatred of the enemy. Ample *opportunity* for the assaults had to do with the location of the prisoners' living quarters, that we referred to as the *far corner* of the compound.

For obvious reasons the prisoners' living quarters were situated at the edge of the square-shaped compound, and the Quonset-hut cells were aligned in such a way that the prisoners could not easily observe the compound buildings from inside the Quonset huts.

The particulars of the execution of the prisoners upon the completion of their interrogation were discussed among the seven interrogators speaking in Korean, in order that the American support troops not be a part to these communications, as support troops did not possess Top Secret Clearances, nor did they have a need to know.

However both the interrogators and the support troops were well aware that on the afternoon of the typing of the Final Interrogation Summary there would be no valid reason to extend for even a day the time for the prisoner to remain on the compound. Or, for that matter, to remain alive.

This schedule of executing a North Korean spy within hours of the completion of his interrogation may seem to a layman, especially an American, to be out of step with legal due process, because of our appeals processes both civilian and military being at the core of our system of jurisprudence.

However South Korean law mandated the *automatic* execution of any North Korean spy captured in South Korea, from which there was *no right of appeal*. His fate was sealed on the day of his capture and no amount of cooperation could ever change this law or lessen this penalty.

I have never been a morbidly-curious person. However this was to be the execution of my first prisoner and I naturally wanted to know what to expect. So a few days before I wrote and twixed to G-2 my Final Interrogation Summary I ended up after supper one night walking from the mess hall inside the headquarters building to the *club*, a building that housed – because the 502 was such a small base – both the EM (Enlisted Men's) Club and the Officers' Club - with several of the interrogators.

"Within a few days I'll be writing my Final Interrogation Summary, as Col. Kim and I have gotten about as much out of the prisoner as possible," I said to no one in particular. "Anyone care to fill me in on what happens next?"

"Let's go into the club, you guys," said one of the older interrogators. "For the price of a round of beers, Provost here will get the scoop on the prisoner's last night at the 502." The *scoop* turned out to be an eye-opener. I was mesmerized by his explanation, almost to the point that I regretted having asked the question.

"The first thing you have to understand Provost, is the degree of hatred the North Koreans and South Koreans have for one another," he began. "And just as we're trying to break up North Korean espionage rings in South Korea, the North Koreans in Pyongyang are searching for South Korean spies in North Korea. We're still at war, nine years into an Armistice."

"How does this relate to my prisoner?" I asked.

"The M.P. guards are just aching to beat these prisoners to death, but they know they can't touch them," he said. "However the prisoner has been scheduled for execution and the Korean M.P.s will come that same night in a paddy wagon, that is enclosed so there is no way for the prisoner to escape during the trip from the 502 to the Wall at Inchon. However during the trip two of the M.P.s are alone with the prisoner inside the enclosed paddy wagon."

"I understand what you mean," I said. "Nobody at the 502 will ever see the prisoner again, so there is no one that the prisoner can complain to. What happens when they arrive at the Wall?"

"It's all over within a few minutes," said the interrogator. "About midway between here and Inchon there is out in a field a rock wall. There is no formal ceremony. The M.P.s just stand the prisoner up against the wall and form a three-man firing squad. Then the execution is carried out. Or this has always been our understanding of the procedure."

"Have any of the interrogators ever witnessed an execution?" I asked.

"A few of us have," he said. "Why, are you interested yourself?"

"No, thank you," I quickly responded. "If I interrogated a prisoner for months and got to know him well, I'd likely have nightmares for years afterwards if I witnessed his execution. But thanks all the same."

I never did witness the execution of a North Korean prisoner. And I have never regretted this decision.

And despite this I still had nightmares.

"Think about it for a moment Provost," said one of the older interrogators. "If we complain to the colonel, what is he going to do?"

"I would admit, not much."

"You are correct, except that the Korean M.P.s will know the Americans have complained," he said. "And it comes right down to what would we do if we were South Koreans and the North Koreans had infiltrated from across the border with the intention of murdering us?"

"I suppose I would feel the same," I admitted, wondering how many of these muffled cries of pain had been coming from *my* prisoner.

Was this yet another Korean problem with a Korean solution? I wondered.

Saying Farewell

Finally the prisoner's last day of interrogation arrived. It was a general review of the two months of daily interrogations. I found it difficult looking the Communist espionage agent in the eye.

Instead I reached into my jacket pocket and withdrew the two Hershey chocolate bars. I pushed them across the table to him.

"Put these in your pocket and eat them when you get back to your cell," I said.

"Thank you," he said, picking up the candy bars and putting them into his trouser pocket. Then he looked me in the eyes and added, almost as an afterthought,

"Thank you for everything you have done for me."

Suddenly I knew that he knew.

Realizing that he sensed this likely would be the night of his execution, I stood and extended my right hand across the table. He stood and we shook hands. I'll never forget that moment. Perhaps I wasn't cut out for this job after all?

Col. Kim and I agreed that my first interrogation had been a successful one, even though truth be told a portion of the material gleaned from the prisoner was cumulative in nature. However we were harvesters of information. The analysts back at G-2 in the Pentagon would make decisions as to how our data fitted into the North Koreans' overall grand scheme of their espionage network in South Korea. I was definitely heartened by Col. Kim's compliment. He had made my first interrogation meaningful.

Our task was to continue with my second prisoner the following morning. However the sleep I acquired the night of my first prisoner's execution lasted one or two hours at best.

I framed in my mind the prisoner inside a closed wire paddy wagon as it sped through the darkness along the road to Inchon, and envisioned the execution being carried out in front of a cinder block and rock wall. The abject surrealism of it all was ponderous and quite palpable. Never in my life had I felt so indecisive. That moment has been with me forever. Always will be.

Indecisive. And singularly quite helpless. I realized that I had some inner problems to work out in my mind before I could settle in and begin to accept that a part of my duties would quickly become a fact of life and an integral part of my psyche.

Without this acceptance how could I ever hope to come to terms with the knowledge that every prisoner I interrogated during the ensuing months would end his life standing bruised and battered in front of a rock wall situated along the lonely Seoul-to-Inchon road just after midnight.

I recalled eating with the interrogators in the 502 mess hall when I was the feature writer for the *Stars & Stripes*. As Jon Powell had introduced me to some of the interrogators I couldn't help but notice the small bottles filled with a chalky white liquid resting on the dining table near their plates.

Upon inquiring as to the purpose of this liquid, Powell had informed me that every prisoner interrogator, due to the daily stresses and demands of the job, sooner than later developed ulcers. Thus in a subtle way I had been warned.

There is no question in my mind but that my empathy for these doomed North Korean spies stemmed in large degree from my own life's travails. A discussion of my unfortunate experiences as an orphan in Oxford Orphanage from the ages of seven to seventeen is similar in many ways to the plight of these North Korean espionage agents and minders.

First of all neither I nor the communist spies volunteered for the unfortunate circumstances in which we found ourselves. We had absolutely no control over our fate. This sense of despair has been with me ever since, and I'm certain will follow me to my gibbet.

Chapter 18

◇◇◇◇◇

Investigating the Communist Economy

Early on in our interrogation of my first prisoner, one day the Korean waitresses served us Americans oranges. Not particularly craving an orange at the moment, I carried the fruit back to the I.C. and placed it on the corner of the table. Perhaps the prisoner would like the orange for dessert, because the prisoners were served Korean food exclusively. And besides, thought I, who doesn't like oranges?

I still believe "dessert" was an invention of Southern mothers used to entice small children into eating all that squash, okra and turnips that the mothers piled on the kids' plate. Of course I could be wrong. But I don't think so.

Col. Kim and I were already seated at the rectangular table when the M.P. opened the door to the I.R. and motioned for the prisoner to enter and sit across from the colonel and myself.

After we three were seated I picked up the bright orange-colored orange and placed the fruit on the table in front of the prisoner.

"I brought this for you. Go right ahead and eat it," I encouraged.

"I would rather not eat it," said the prisoner.

"But don't you like oranges?" asked the naïve young American soldier.

"No," offered Col. Kim. "This is the first orange he has even seen. Oranges don't grow in Korea, either north or south."

"But he probably would like it," I said.

"Let's try something," said the colonel, reaching into his pocket and pulling out a small jackknife.

"May I cut the orange into four parts?" he asked.

"Why certainly," I responded.

The colonel did so, then returned the jackknife to his pocket. He placed one of the four parts on the table in front of the prisoner. He then picked up one of the wedges, peeled it and ate the fruit.

I followed suit. When the prisoner observed me swallowing the orange, he smiled, then picked up the orange quarter, peeled it, and took a bite.

And abruptly made the universal face young children make to show their mothers that they do not like the taste of something. I looked at Col. Kim in puzzlement.

"Koreans crave things that are sweet, like sugar, Hershey's chocolate bars and Juicy Fruit gum," said Col. Kim. But to this prisoner the orange has a bitter taste, so he won't eat it."

"What about bananas, peaches, pears, lemons and apples?" I asked the colonel.

"I assure you that this North Korean peasant has never seen a banana, a peach, a lemon or a pear," he responded. "And the only apples he has seen grow wild in the country. A fruit is a luxury to a North Korean, and the concept of *dessert* is foreign to him."

"This is very interesting," I said. "What about milk, butter, cheese and ice cream?"

"None of these foods exist in North Korea, and there aren't a lot of them even in South Korea."

"And why is this?" I asked quizzically.

"During the year and three months you spent traveling around South Korea for the *Stars & Stripes*, how many milk cows did you see?"

What an odd question, I thought. However following a few moments of reflection I believed I had the answer to Col. Kim's question. The answer was *zero*.

"Why, I don't recall seeing any cows. I suppose I assumed they were inside the barn being milked."

"No, you didn't recall seeing any milk cows because there were no milk cows in North Korea or South Korea. Still aren't," he said. "Therefore most Koreans have never tasted milk, butter, cheese or ice cream."

"It seems as though most Koreans, especially the children, like chocolate candy and chewing gum," I said.

"This is true, except that to a Korean, chewing gum *is* candy."

"What do you mean?"

"Americans chew a stick of gum for awhile, then spit it out. However this concept is difficult for a Korean to comprehend. Thus when a Korean tires of chewing the gum, he simply swallows it, just as he would swallow the piece of candy."

At this time Col. Kim excused himself. He walked down the hall, then returned carrying four thick notebooks, that he placed on the table. The notebooks were printed in English. He sat down, selected one of the notebooks, and placed the other three to the side.

"What do we have here?" I asked.

"These notebooks are very important," he said, opening the notebook to a random page. "After we finish interrogating the prisoner, and if we have time on our hands while we wait for the next prisoner, we begin interrogating him concerning various aspects of civilian and military life."

"For example?" I said.

"Nearly every North Korean agent or minder entered their espionage system from the military. We need to know the makeup of his unit, whether the soldiers were well-fed or not, whether their troops were short on heating fuel during the winter, etc."

"What is done with this data?"

"It's twixed on to G-2 in Washington, where it is collated with similar data from around North Korea. Examples are as follows:"

Are there chronic food, uniform and ammunition shortages, especially during the winter months? Military? Civilian?

What is the morale of the military units?

Is AWOL a big worry? Desertion? Suicide?

What are the troops told about American soldiers? About Americans in general?

"As we continue our interrogations you'll see what appears to be redundancies in our questioning. But keep in mind that this is intentional," said Col. Kim.

"And the purpose of this?" I asked quizzically.

"Because the analysts back at the Pentagon need to be made aware of any *changes* in civilian and military life inside North Korea," he explained.

"For example?"

"Assume that gasoline is rationed, which of course it is. So one prisoner reports that the gasoline ration was three gallons to each automobile per week," he explained.

"Then your next prisoner, in response to this same question six months later, reports that the gasoline ration is now *one* gallon per week. This would be a significant change indicating a rapidly worsening economy. And these civilian changes at the same time are also felt in the military. So if gasoline is rationed in civilian cars, this will also be reflected in military vehicles."

This data is important, according to Col. Kim, because ninety percent of intelligence the United States gathers on North Korea comes from seven prisoner interrogators toiling away inside the 502 I.C. in Seoul. The other ten percent of intelligence comes from the aerial photographs taken by pilots flying the U2 at 60,000 feet above North Korea. Thus the analysts need data on military *and civilian* life.

Given this state of affairs it is easy to understand why we seven prisoner interrogators felt the constant pressure to produce results.

The name given to this form of questions was called "trends," or "patterns." At first blush these questions might appear to be innocuous. However in the aggregate they established a pattern of the health of the North Korean economy.

Also helpful was the fact that because these questions were a mixture of military and civilian subjects, the prisoner could find no reason to lie to the interrogator. Thus this form of questioning told us a lot about the state of the economy, and this in turn told us about the state of the North Korean military's readiness.

First-hand accounts from apprehended communist agents and minders consistently painted a grim picture of a backward nation with little hope for improvement in the future, and of harsh winters in which soldiers fared better than the civilian population.

We interrogators never witnessed the enemy agents eating their meals. During our lunch break at 12:00 noon we walked over to the mess hall while the prisoners were returned to their Quonset hut cells. Their meals were brought to them by the South Korean Army M.P.s.

However Col. Kim informed me that to a man, every captured communist agent or minder appeared to be undernourished when he was brought to the 502 compound.

Upon my return to Korea following a year at the Defense Language Institute I found myself in a unique position to *fill in the blanks* so to speak concerning the Big Book, that had to do with investigating the communist economy, that over time offered glimpses of the military readiness using civilian life as a starting point for my analyses.

With this data the analysts back at G-2 in the Pentagon should be able to determine the North Korean Army's ability to conduct combat operations including sustaining itself.

Chapter 19

◇◇◇◇◇

My Second Prisoner:
Fate of the Wounded Enemy Agent

Quite often we at the 502 would receive a captured North Korean espionage *agent*, not a minder, who had been apprehended by a South Korean Army patrol shortly after wading ashore along the craggy East Sea coastline.

And on this particular occasion, upon discovery by the army patrol, the two minders had fled. When captured the agent was carrying a map of South Korea and $30,000 in hundred-dollar bills together with $15,000 in Korean *won*, secreted inside a wide cloth money belt.

And he was in a lot of pain.

During the firefight the abandoned agent had dropped his money belt and fled into the thick woods. A jacketed round from an M-1 rifle had struck the agent in the upper thigh, ripping out part of the muscle and rendering him crippled.

However rather than transport the enemy agent to a hospital, the ROK soldiers staunched the flow of blood and delivered him to the 502, right on our doorstep. Literally.

When the ROK Army soldiers arrived at the 502 with the wounded prisoner in tow, one of the other interrogators and I were on our way from the headquarters building to the I.C. (Interrogation Center). The ROK Army Jeep stopped in front of the I.C. and we asked the soldiers why the man was sprawled across the back seat of the Jeep.

When they explained who was the wounded man, we walked back to the headquarters building and explained the situation. The major told us to drive the man to the Eighth U.S. Army dispensary in Seoul.

We placed the agonizing prisoner in a Jeep and rushed him to the dispensary at Yongsan. An x-ray of the left thigh showed that the powerful M1 round had also struck bone, driving shards of bone into muscle.

This enemy agent was at the same time the Eighth U.S. Army physician's *patient*. After examining the wound and the x-rays the physician shook his head and spoke evenly.

"This man must have his left leg amputated. I can dig out the bone fragments, but if we don't amputate, gangrene may well set in, and he could even lose his life."

This brief discussion had taken place in the presence of the prisoner, who, while lying prone on the bed in the dispensary could tell by all those present pointing down at his left leg every time they made a statement or asked a question that he – or better still the useless left leg – was the center of attention.

Suddenly he became quite agitated and spoke in a raised voice. The physician, who of course did not speak Korean, looked back and forth between me and the other interrogator who had come along in case someone else at the dispensary needed a translator.

"Provost, the doctor here is not cleared, so let's be careful what we say," he said.

"I understand," I responded.

"What's going on?" asked the physician.

"Who is this man anyway?" again gesturing with his hand toward the prisoner.

"No use in both of us getting into trouble," I said to him. "Why don't you step out into the hall for just a moment."

Without comment he exited the room, leaving the doctor and me standing at the foot of the bed. I spoke to the prisoner who nodded his head in response. Then I turned to the doctor, who was a major in the U.S. Army Medical Corps.

"Sir, the man who just left the room and I are prisoner interrogators at the 502 Military Intelligence Battalion out on the Osan Highway in Yungdung-po. The ROK Army captured this spy early this morning.

"I wondered why those two American M.P.s were standing out in the hallway," he said, slowly nodding his head in understanding.

"In order to be privy to anything the prisoner says, you are supposed to have a Top Secret Security Clearance and a need to know. As the prisoner's physician you don't have the clearance but definitely have the need to know his medical condition," I said.

"Please understand that I am in violation of my security clearance just by explaining this to you. So I really need to keep this conversation between us."

"I understand," said the major.

"I'm going to explain to the prisoner that you are going to have to amputate his left leg."

The major listened intently as I explained to the North Korean that in order to save his life the physician would have to cut off his leg at the hip. This comment elicited an instant anguished wailing.

"What did he say?" asked the major worriedly.

"He asked why you need to cut off his leg since he was going to be executed soon anyway."

The physician was taken aback by the abrupt question, turning to me for an explanation.

"This man is a North Korean spy who was shot up over on the coast when he was captured," I said. "And he is correct. As a spy, the penalty is execution. But he has critical information that we need as soon as possible."

"And are you and your friend out in the hall both prisoner interrogators?"

"Yes we are. I asked him to wait outside. In the event I catch hell for telling you all this, both of us won't be thrown in the stockade."

"Don't worry Provost," he said smiling. "Your secret is safe with me."

"What would happen if you did not amputate?" I asked.

"He is likely going to end up crippled. But if I cleaned up the wound, we might be able to save the leg. No doubt it would be touch-and-go for several weeks."

"If we keep him out at the 502, could you send a medic out once a day to change his bandages?" I asked.

"This would not be a problem," said the major. He paused, then added, "Don't worry Provost. Your secret is safe with me. It's just that you don't seem to fit the mold of what I always pictured a prisoner interrogator to look like."

"I can't say that being a prisoner interrogator has always been fun," I said. "However it certainly has been interesting."

The other interrogator, the two M.P.s and I waited around for about an hour while the physician plucked the bone fragments from the prisoner's thigh, cleaned the wound and placed a splint on his leg. Then we loaded the prisoner into our Jeep and returned to the 502. Not that the prisoner would be likely to get much use of it but the physician threw in a pair of wooden crutches for good measure. Yeah, as though the crippled communist spy were going to take an evening stroll around the 502 *campus*.

An Offer the Prisoner Couldn't Refuse

Because Col. Kim and I had not begun interrogating our next prisoner, we were assigned to interrogate the wounded enemy agent.

The Korean workers brought two chairs and a small table into the Quonset-hut cell and we questioned the prisoner while he was lying prone on his metal cot.

As the prisoner in his debilitated, weakened state would be expected to tire quickly, we interrogated him for three hours each day, from 8:00 a.m. – 11:00 a.m., then took on another prisoner from 1:00 p.m. – 4:00 p.m.

We began our interrogation of the prisoner the following morning. I asked Col. Kim to make the following point to the prisoner:

The army doctor recommended that we amputate the prisoner's left leg. However Col. Kim and I pleaded with the doctor not to do so in order to spare the prisoner the indignity that the surgery would bring.

I was singularly impressed. This poor Korean realized he would be executed within so many months. Yet his biggest fear was losing face among the Korean guards by losing his leg! Gutsy, he was.

Thus Col. Kim struck a deal with the prisoner. As long as the prisoner answered our questions truthfully, Col. Kim and the American would ensure that the doctor would not amputate his leg.

And I might add that as far as Col. Kim and I were concerned, the prisoner kept his end of the bargain. We extracted valuable information from the prisoner. However after two months passed it came time to type my Final Interrogation Summary.

South Korean Law Takes Over

After Col. Kim and I had written our Final Interrogation Summary, stating in the conclusion that we believed the prisoner possessed no additional information of value, the South Korean military commander arranged for the execution of the prisoner that would take place at *The Wall*, located approximately halfway between Seoul and Inchon, or about twenty miles west of the 502. The area was referred to as simply *The Wall at Inchon* because the rock wall was the only permanent structure at the site, according to Col. Kim.

In South Korea during the 1960s, whenever possible the army transported its prisoners in what we Americans referred to as "paddy wagons," for security purposes. The vehicle was somewhat larger than a Jeep, and consisted of a cab and an enclosed container, part of the side walls containing a wire window for purposes of ventilation.

Paddy wagons were used because there was no way for the handcuffed prisoner to escape, as opposed to an open-air Jeep.

According to Col. Kim and a few of the interrogators, there was no definite time for the paddy wagon to arrive at the main gate of the 502 to collect the prisoner. Usually, everyone seemed to agree, this time could be anywhere between midnight and daybreak.

However it seemed the unfortunate prisoner always knew. Perhaps the Korean M.P.s had told the prisoner his time was up. Or else he sensed his interrogators had fewer questions for him. But the prisoner always knew.

"Will they come for me tonight?" asked the prisoner from his bunk inside his Quonset-hut cell, where we had interrogated him during the two months he had been our prisoner.

The prisoners were well aware of what went on inside the fenced-in compound that was the 502. After dark the only persons present in that far corner were the prisoners and the South Korean Army guards, who were M.P.s. And the wounded enemy agent was astute enough to see the writing on the metal wall of his Quonset-hut cell concerning his fate.

"Unfortunately they don't tell us when they do certain things around here," I answered honestly. "But what would you want me to do for you?"

"The North Korean Army officers did not tell me the truth," he said.

"How did they lie to you?" I asked quizzically.

"They said you would torture me. But you are an American and have treated me well," he said. "And for this I thank you."

From his prone position on his bunk he extended his right hand up to me. We shook hands, and I could see the tears welling up in his eyes. He knew his time had come.

"Could you come to see me before they take me away?" His subdued voice was almost pleading.

I turned to Col. Kim.

"I don't see why not," said the colonel in English. "I'll tell the army commander and he'll set a definite time for the M.P.s to come for him. We're not breaking any rules because we have completed our interrogation of the prisoner."

At supper that same night one of the Korean waitresses stopped by my table. She leaned down and spoke softly.

"They are coming at ten tonight."

"Thank you," I said.

I arrived at the prisoner's Quonset-hut cell at 9:30 p.m. The M.P.s had been informed that I was coming and one of them unlocked the cell.

"Go ahead and visit with him," said the M.P. "When the paddy wagon gets here they will be in a hurry and they can't wait. I hope you understand."

The prisoner still was unable to stand. So I sat at the small interrogation table in his cell while he lay on his metal cot.

I began by asking him more about the village where he had been born, about his friends and family, anything to take his mind off his fate.

However I could readily see the fear in his eyes and hear the apprehension in his voice. But he never cried during the thirty minutes we were waiting for the paddy wagon to give him the ride to his execution. He was one really brave Korean.

The paddy wagon arrived and parked just outside his cell. There were a driver and two men inside the paddy wagon, all three M.P.s. They got out and approached me in the darkness.

"Are you Provost?" asked one of them.

"Yes I am," I replied.

"Do you need any more time?" asked a second Korean M.P. "We're in no hurry."

"No, he's ready to go. You'll have to carry him to the paddy wagon because he still cannot walk. Please go easy on him."

Two of the South Korean M.P.s assisted the prisoner in climbing up into the paddy wagon. Just before he was lifted up he extended his right hand and I shook it.

When the two M.P.s had deposited the prisoner inside the enclosed bay of the paddy wagon, they climbed in with him. When they closed and secured the rear door of the vehicle I turned to the driver.

"This prisoner is crippled and therefore can't defend himself," I said. "I know what happens when you get the doomed prisoners in the paddy wagon. So please, as a favor to me, don't hurt him."

The M.P. passed my request on to the other two and they loaded the prisoner into the paddy wagon. I only hope that they had honored my request.

Chapter 20

◇◇◇◇◇

My Third Prisoner: A Political Mystery Who Was James William Fulbright?

And even more important, what did he have to do with Company A, 502 Military Intelligence Battalion, in 1965?

The fastest typist in the 502 wasn't even *in* the 502. He was one of the two American CIA agents. However I was the second fastest typist on the compound. For fifteen months prior to leaving the *Stars & Stripes* for greener pastures i.e., to study Korean for a year at the Defense Language Institute, located in the California seaside resort town of Monterey, I had been the newspaper's (circulation 45,000) only feature writer, and was enjoying every minute of it.

At the *Stars & Stripes* each reporter typed his own stories, so I was typing at least part of each day. For some unknown reason, when I arrived at the 502 I found that several of the interrogators were still using the old hunt-and-peck method of typing. Just like at the newspaper, each interrogator was responsible for typing his own Interrogation Summaries. So I offered to help out so long as I had nothing planned after one of the interrogators and two American M.P.s were on their way to the Eighth U.S. Army "Twix Center" with the valise of Summaries.

However my offer to assist with the typing was neither totally altruistic nor entirely selfless. Because in assisting with the typing I was able to read the Interrogation Summaries of some of the other six interrogators. And many of the summaries were quite interesting. I discovered after a few months that some of the interrogators were naturally better at their job than were others, but all six appeared to be dedicated to the work they were performing. At no time did an interrogator report that he had felt a need to threaten a prisoner.

James William Fulbright (1905-1995) was a United States Senator who represented Arkansas from January 1945 until his resignation in

December 1974. Of interest to our story is the fact that Senator Fulbright was the longest serving Chairman in the history of the Senate Foreign Relations Committee, that included the period 1964-65 when I served as an interrogator at the 502.

Now it had always been the understanding of the seven interrogators that the prisoner would be picked up from the compound sometime between 12:00 midnight and 6:00 a.m. The three Korean Army M.P.s would place the doomed prisoner inside the oversized paddy wagon and drive west on the Seoul-Inchon road to the execution site located approximately twenty miles west of the 502. That the prisoner could be granted a reprieve from *anyone* was unheard of on the 502 compound.

Did someone know something we didn't know? Were they keeping us out of the loop?

On the day following the execution of the luckless, crippled agent, at 8:00 a.m. I met Col. Kim at the I.C. to ask about any new arrivals. When the question was answered in the negative, I asked the officer on duty if I could borrow a Jeep and make a short run to Yongsan.

I needed to drive in to Eighth U.S. Army Headquarters to the Bank of America located near the large PX. We were paid in cash near the first of each month, and because I neither drank nor smoked I deposited most of my $1300 salary into my account at Bank of America.

As mentioned previously the officers likely had been instructed by the colonel to allow the seven interrogators any reasonable amount of time away from the compound between interrogations, and we referred to this freedom as *mental health days*. In other words I didn't have to rush to Yongsan, then rush back to the 502.

So I didn't. Rush back, that is. I went to the bank, made my deposit, tarried for an hour or so inside the giant PX, then stopped in at a small ice cream shop for a large chocolate milk shake. And then I had another, for good measure.

I drove back inside the main gate at 12:30, and the American M.P. held up his hand.

"Provost, the colonel wants to see you over at the I.C. He's got you and Col. Kim a new *customer*."

Inside the I.C. our colonel and Col. Kim were waiting for me. The new "customer" was seated alone at the table inside our interrogation room, being watched over by a Korean M.P. standing at the door. We viewed the prisoner through the 2-way mirror.

"He looks awfully composed to have just recently been captured," observed Col. Kim. And I agreed. This alone seemed odd.

Col. Kim and I reiterated our standard introduction to the new prisoner. My partner explained to him that he, Col. Kim, had the "pull" with the South Korean authorities that would forego the prisoner's execution in favor of a 20-year prison sentence, provided the prisoner cooperated and answered all questions truthfully. I sat still and nodded imperceptibly my agreement with Col. Kim's blatant deception. My subtle reinforcement tended to win the day. His story follows.

The prisoner was a 35-year-old major in the North Korean Army. He commanded an artillery training regiment at a large base forty kilometers east of Pyongyang, the capital of North Korea.

I had figured a way to test the prisoner's story. Following Basic Infantry Training at Ft. Jackson, South Carolina in the summer of 1961, I had undergone eight weeks of Advanced Artillery Training, specifically in a 105mm Howitzer battery, at Ft. Sill. If it were true that he was a major and commanded an artillery training regiment, surely he should have known the rudimentary operation of the 105mm Howitzer.

"What can you tell us about the operation of the American Army's 105mm Howitzer?" I asked abruptly, expecting the question to confuse the prisoner.

Didn't do it however. The North Korean Army officer rattled off the specifications of the 105mm Howitzer like he had invented the weapon, even praising it for its accuracy.

When I next asked him about the U.S. Army's larger 155mm Howitzer, again without any hesitation he gave us the weapon's specifications quite accurately. So much for his veracity. Sure convinced me anyway.

Col. Kim and I followed our standard interrogation format. He was an *agent*. He had been charged to deliver the American and South Korean money to a safehouse in a small fishing village south of Sokcho, South Korea. Further orders would be given to the prisoner by the North Korean spy waiting inside the safehouse.

The agent realized he was at the mercy of the two minders sent along to protect him. He sensed however, although no one in Pyongyang had informed him, that if ever the 3-man team came under attack the two minders would kill him to prevent his capture.

The agent also was aware that the two minders carried no money or food, and he sensed that neither could read a road map because only the agent had received a map before the fishing trawler set out from Wonsan under the cover of darkness.

With all these fears in mind, as soon as the agent had an opportunity he slipped away in the darkness. This was the last he had seen of the minders. At daybreak he realized he was surrounded by about a dozen South Korean Army troops, and surrendered.

We interrogated the major for about six weeks. At the end of this period Col. Kim and I met inside the I.C. at the end of the day. We agreed that he had given us all the pertinent information he had, and I made plans to submit my Final Interrogation Summary in two days. The mission planners back in Pyongyang had informed the major that he would receive his orders from the North Korean cell ringleader inside the safehouse, and because he never reached the safehouse he had no useful information in that regard.

At 8:00 a.m. the following morning we began our last day of interrogation. At 10:00 a.m. one of the U.S. Army M.P.s knocked on the door of our interrogation room. I opened the door to see the M.P. holding an official-looking envelope in his hand. He handed it to me.

"This just came in the mail, Provost. The colonel said for you to type and sign your Final Interrogation Summary, and bring it to the office."

The envelope contained three letters. On the first week of his capture the major had asked for a sheet of plain copy paper. The colonel granted his request. The prisoner wrote a letter in Korean, but asked that it be translated into English and delivered to *Senator William Fulbright* of the U.S. Senate. We did not see the English translation of that letter. At the time, we interrogators looked at one another seeking an answer to this question: How in blazes does this prisoner know Senator James William Fulbright?

So we just continued our interrogation. The second letter received that last morning was the translation of the letter the major wrote in Korean.

The letter was addressed to Senator Fulbright. It argued that the prisoner should not be executed because he had been sent by North Korean officials to deliver money. He argued that because he was not armed, either with a gun or knife, this fact supported his contention that he had no intention of harming anyone. He was making his best argument for extenuating circumstances.

The third letter really captured everyone's attention. It was printed on the official stationary of the Senate of the United States. In short the letter was addressed to the Commander of U.S. Forces Korea. It named the prisoner of war specifically, and requested that any action on his case be delayed pending a hearing. The letter listed no specific date for this hearing.

I knew two things to be true from reading the senator's letter. First of all I assumed the letter was our colonel's way of ordering us to suspend our interrogation until the colonel could answer the letter. However nothing was said in this regard.

The second thing we interrogators knew was that because the prisoner, like those who came before and after him, had by law been sentenced to death the instant he placed his foot south of the Demilitarized Zone (DMZ), the only person who had the authority to stay his execution was a high-ranking military officer, either American or South Korean.

Officially the prisoner was the property of the South Korean Army, not the U.S. Army. He, the prisoner, was simply "on loan" to the 502 for the purpose of interrogation. Furthermore within an hour I would be filing my Final Interrogation Summary.

Because the prisoner was mine *and* Col. Kim's, I asked Col. Kim what would be his advice.

"Provost, this situation has occurred before. All I can tell you is that the prisoner will be taken away in a paddy wagon tonight and will be executed tonight."

"I fully understand your position, Col. Kim. Furthermore I agree with it," I said. "So what should we do?"

"I think you and I should stay out of any argument between your colonel in the 502 and my superior officer. But I have a duty to report this to my superiors. They will know what is best to do. May I take these three letters and show them to him?" The Korean military maintained an office on the 502 compound.

"I'll wait for you back at the I.C.," I said, handing him the three letters.

About an hour later Col. Kim returned from the Korean Army's office.

"My commanding officer said the problem should be cleared up by tomorrow afternoon," said the colonel.

I filed my Final Interrogation Summary in the office along with the three letters, without comment. I assumed that when Col. Kim showed the three letters to his commanding officer, the latter would contact our 502 colonel and the two senior officers would reach some accommodation.

There were two conflicting considerations in this regard. Col. Kim appeared certain that the South Korean junta who controlled the nation in 1964-1965, following the bloodless coup of May 16, 1961, would not make an exception to South Korean law, especially because the fact the North Korean major was unarmed was not occasioned by any altruistic reasons on his part. If given a choice the North Korean agent certainly would have been carrying at least two loaded pistols, possibly three, if for no other reason than to protect himself against two trigger-happy minders. The major knew the score.

Anyway Col. Kim and I had filed our Final Interrogation Summaries along with the three letters, so we were, to use the vernacular, "out of the picture."

At supper an hour or so later we interrogators were speculating on the fate of the prisoner. The South Korean Army showed a great deal of obsequious deference to the U.S. Army, historically-speaking. Would the Koreans relent and spare the North Korean major's life, at least until they could convene a hearing?

Unfortunately for the major, apparently not.

After a week or so passed and the smoke had cleared from this fiasco, a thing or two bothered me still. Because the South Korean M.P.s would naturally take great satisfaction in informing the prisoners of their approaching execution date, usually in those last few days of interrogation they would become somewhat quieter, as though deep in thought. Or worry.

However the major showed not the slightest signs of distress, even as he was being escorted back to his Quonset hut cell at 4:00 p.m., and did not appear eager to say any final goodbyes or thank yous. Did he think he knew something we didn't know?

The morning following the *letters* incident of the previous afternoon, I met Col. Kim outside the I.C. We greeted one another, then entered the building and walked back to our interrogation room, Col. Kim following me. As I opened the door to the room, Col. Kim answered the question that was on my lips but yet unspoken, i.e., "Where's the prisoner?"

"He's not here, Provost. As soon as it became dark, the paddy wagon came for him. Korean law makes no exceptions for North Korean spies. He was executed at 8:30 p.m."

During the next few weeks several puzzling thoughts assailed my mind. Why had I not heard from our 502 colonel since the major's execution? How had the prisoner known about a specific American Senator? The only possible tie-in between the prisoner and the senator was that during this time Senator Fulbright became known for his opposition to American involvement in the Vietnam War. So what?

We interrogators remained puzzled over the incident. Two days later I began interrogating my fourth prisoner in just over six months. Was I going to set some sort of record for communist spies executed?

The person most surprised by the outcome of this case must have been the North Korean major the night he heard the familiar whine of the paddy wagon's engine as it drove up and parked in front of his Quonset-hut cell. At the time I ended my tour of duty less than a year later I still had not heard a plausible explanation to the following questions: How did the North Korean Army major know of Senator William Fulbright? Second, what was it he *thought* he knew that gave him the confidence that he would not be executed on the last day of his interrogation? We'll never know. Strange, to say the least.

Researching the Troublesome Case

In researching this puzzle I came upon several interesting aspects of the life and politics of this influential elder statesman. He was a

Southern Democrat and staunch segregationist, one of the signers of the *Southern Manifesto*.

Senator Fulbright became chairman of the Senate Foreign Relations Committee, where he held several televised hearings on America's involvement in the Vietnam War. In 1966, the year after the North Korean officer became a prisoner at the 502, the senator published *The Arrogance of Power*, in which he expressed his opposition to the war in Vietnam.

In attempting to find a nexus between a powerful U.S. senator's opposition to the Vietnam War and a North Korean espionage agent facing execution as a communist spy in South Korea however, I could not envision any set of circumstances in which the North Korean army officer could expect a powerful U.S. senator to demand that the South Korean government spare his life.

To this day the case remains a puzzle.

Chapter 21

◇◇◇◇◇

Had I Bitten Off More Than I Could Chew?

It was at this very moment that I questioned whether I was well-suited for this high-pressure job, or was completely out of my element.

However these doubts arose not from a qualification or training point of view. No, even at the young age of 25 I felt confident in my ability to match wits with a communist espionage agent seated a mere three-to-four feet away and by guile and wit to draw out of him the details of his mission. No, from an operational standpoint I believed I would become an excellent prisoner interrogator. However,…

Being emotionally and psychologically prepared to interrogate a North Korean espionage agent when both the agent and you are acutely aware that his life expectancy suddenly becomes measured in months – and an excruciatingly few of those – is a different matter entirely. And this would be my second prisoner to be executed in a span of less than four months.

What concerned me initially was my discovery, upon the beginning of the interrogation of my first prisoner, an agent, that the 28-year-old North Korean Army Private with possibly a sixth grade or less education, *had not volunteered* for this mission but had been selected solely because of his accuracy with a rifle.

And this was true even though he had been informed that his three-man team – only the two minders being armed, mind you – would not stand a chance in a firefight with a well-armed South Korean shore patrol.

During the wounded communist agent's two months of interrogation inside his cell, we questioned him only for approximately three hours each morning. His desire not to have his left leg amputated led to constant pain, this pain subsiding as the days passed, though never to the point of allowing him to walk or even to stand up from a prone position.

"Did your superiors explain to you what would happen to you if you were captured in South Korea?"

This question was posed to each captured minder or agent early on in the beginning of interrogation. The answer:

"Yes, I was told that I would be interrogated and then executed."

This answer was elicited from each frightened enemy agent or minder. And this response from the North Korean officers was correct in every sense. However it was the interrogator's job to make the doomed prisoner believe that there was indeed a light at the end of this dark tunnel.

If the 502 had had a motto, it would have been "Hurry, time's a-wasting." Everything we did was urgent, and one thing the few officers insisted on – because some antsy analyst back at G-2 inside the Pentagon had insisted on it – was that all interrogations cease at 4:00 p.m. in order to type our Daily Interrogation Summaries and have them delivered to the Twix Center at the Eighth U.S. Army Headquarters in Yongsan by 6:00 p.m.

Thus it was the interrogator's job to take as long as it took to convince the prisoner that his superiors' claim that his life would end standing in front of a three-man South Korean Army firing squad was patently false, because his fate was definitely in his own hands. The message was clear:

If you answer truthfully our questions, you will not be harmed. You will spend many years in a South Korean prison. But you will not be executed.

In the United States the Supreme Court has consistently upheld the right of police officers to lie to suspects in order to gain an advantage in criminal interrogations.

And it is a certainty that in an espionage case in South Korea the captured enemy agent has no rights of any kind.

Sometimes the feint works and at other times it doesn't. Col. Kim experimented with the possible methods we might use, and finally settled on the following plan.

Col. Kim began by informing the prisoner that he, Col. Kim, had the authority to request the prisoner be granted a reprieve to being executed if he cooperated fully with the interrogators.

As Col. Kim explained the prisoner's (very limited) options I looked straight ahead, nodding silently my agreement with the colonel's blatant, empty lies.

Col. Kim and I agreed that my silent assurances, bolstering his promise to the prisoner, was what cinched the prisoner's cooperation. Maybe so. Maybe not. But I'd like to believe it did.

Sleepless Nights and Little Fears

I have long looked upon worries as what I call "little fears." Put enough of these little fears together and you have the makings of – well, yes, you guessed it – nightmares.

And following the execution of my fourth prisoner, the paratrooper, I sensed the first signs of what I now realize was clinical depression, and it was coming on with a vengeance. This was *the* problem, and it was rapidly becoming *my* problem. Like I owned it or something.

Given the impressive medical advances in psychiatric medicine and research during the past quarter century, words such as *shellshock* have been relegated for use in old World War II and Korean War movies, times during which the all-inclusive term *clinical depression* was just coming into common use in the fields of psychiatry and psychology.

Because South Korean law mandated the automatic execution of all captured North Korean spies, as soon as one of the espionage agents was apprehended and transported to the infamous 502, the prisoner and the interrogator were both acutely aware that the life expectancy of the prisoner was suddenly measured in increments of time shorter than years, usually much shorter.

In addition the interrogator, I or one of my six fellow interrogators, was seated no more than four feet from the prisoner for six hours a day, five days a week for several months.

Given these unusual circumstances then, it would be nigh onto impossible to ignore the prisoner's plight and to not begin to look upon him as a *victim*, especially when the interrogator learns that while confined to that paddy wagon on the dark road to Inchon he is suffering a physical assault at the hands of two South Korean Army M.P.s. Under these circumstances it would be impossible not to experience nightmares on a regular basis, along with shell shock and clinical depression.

I realized the severity of my problem the night following the execution of my second prisoner. As if visions of my first prisoner were not already overtaxing my fragile psyche, suddenly *two* spies were jockeying for the position of who was going to control my sleepless nights.

When I learned from the other interrogators of the abuse of the North Korean prisoners, I kept this revelation to myself simply because I had overheard the conversation in the barracks, and had not been part of the discussion.

After several months passed and I still could not live with knowledge of this abuse, I began to surreptitiously manage to show up in the barracks whenever only a few interrogators were present, hoping that one of the men would draw me into the conversation.

And eventually it happened. As I was sitting on my bunk after supper one night, the interrogator who had picked me up at Kimpo Airport upon my arrival several months earlier, entered the Quonset hut with a friend, who was not an interrogator but was a member of the support personnel. Their discussion centered on their suspected abuse of the prisoners at times *other than* on the night of their execution.

The few officers on the compound realized that the sole purpose of the 502 was to gather information, so they never asked us to perform any chores around the compound, figuring we had enough stress during the daily 6-hour interrogation session.

However they also reasoned that we seven interrogators would not care to be around one another 24 hours a day, so we bunked in the same Quonset huts as did the support troops.

And on this particular night as the two men entered the Quonset hut, seeing me seated on my bunk the interrogator brought me into the conversation.

"Provost, you're the quiet type but you must have an opinion," he began.

"About what?" I asked.

"In the mess hall we were talking about the Korean guards taking advantage of the prisoners. Certainly you've been here long enough to have heard about it."

"I haven't heard any specifics," I lied. "However the prisoners are housed at the far corner of the compound, so who would hear any ruckus from here anyway?"

"Well we all suspect it goes on. But our question is, do we believe that the South Korean *officers* know what's going on?"

"I've given that some thought," I replied. "And I see it this way. The officers hate the North Koreans as much as do the guards, so if the abuse is occurring at the hands of the guards I'm sure the officers would turn the proverbial *blind eye* to the abuse."

This conversation did not ease my mind, but it did let me know that at least one of the interrogators might be open to a discussion on the abuse of the prisoners. At this point I decided to allow a week or so to pass before broaching the subject again.

What I was presented with during the ensuing months amounted to a confirmation of my concerns. And more.

Prisoners were called *Prisoners of War* because this is what they were. The Korean War active fighting ended on July 25, 1953 with the signing of an Armistice. However the Armistice was just that, "a temporary cessation of warfare by mutual agreement." It was by no means a peace treaty. Therefore the North Korean espionage agents who were infiltrated into South Korea along the East Sea were wearing civilian clothes and under the rules of warfare would be classified as *spies* and treated accordingly.

Therefore when a North Korean espionage agent was captured in South Korea the question was not *whether* he would be executed, but *when* the execution would be carried out.

And as mentioned earlier though not discussed in any great detail, this execution date was determined by the American prisoner interrogator. The date was subjective in that *only* the U.S. Army interrogator could sign off on a determination that the prisoner could not offer additional information of value.

South Korean law mandated that spies be executed. There was no such procedural rights that granted an appeal from this death sentence. South Korea? In 1964? No.

And because of this absence of an appeal procedure, the only reason North Korean spies were not summarily executed immediately upon capture was because they were needed at the 502 ASAP if not sooner, for interrogation.

And how long was a North Korean spy held at the 502?

Until one of the seven prisoner interrogators at the 502 signed the Final Interrogation Summary.

When was the execution carried out?

The night following the signing of the Final Interrogation Summary late that same afternoon.

Therefore who determined the prisoner's execution date?

The American interrogator who signed the Final Interrogation Summary. This is the only inescapable conclusion one could reach.

At 4:30 p.m. on the day I signed the Final Interrogation Summary relating to my second prisoner I was in the process of typing the Summary (in triplicate) in the headquarters building, when two of my fellow interrogators entered the typing room.

As I glanced up from my task to acknowledge the two, one of them addressed me.

"How are you doing Provost? And by the way, how are you and Col. Kim coming along with that crippled prisoner?"

There are two basic types of questions in a setting such as this. One question seeks answers, whereas the other is simply a form of polite conversation among friends. His question was of the latter variety.

"Funny you should ask," I stated. "I'm just now typing his Final Interrogation Summary."

"Damn, Provost, what are you trying to do, empty out the cells?" he said laughing.

"Not really," I said. "My first prisoner turned out to be a *minder* not an *agent*. The colonel and I quickly discovered that he really didn't have much to add. And the second prisoner, the wounded agent, isn't going to last much longer. His left leg has become infected for the second time, and his pain medicine is not as effective as when we first started interrogating him. The tremendous pain doesn't allow him to concentrate well on the answers to our questions."

The interrogator's comment concerning Col. Kim and I "emptying out the cells," had unwittingly touched a nerve, but the full import of his remark did not reach my consciousness until a few days later.

However there was indeed a ring of truth to his comment. Here in a span of slightly longer than three months I had personally signed my name to documents which in effect allowed the South Korean Army to execute *two* North Korean espionage agents following a forty-minute drive to a lone rock wall constructed in a field halfway between the 502 in Seoul and the port city of Inchon.

After taking the last half century (1965-2018) to analyze my feelings concerning the plight of these executed North Korean spies, there exists little doubt in my mind that the "closet" empathy I held for these unfortunate souls harked back to my ten years of mental and physical abuse suffered (literally) at the hands of uncaring work supervisors, cottage counselors and teachers. See *Reflections in an Orphan's Eye A Decade at Oxford 1947-1957*, by the author. The 620 page memoir remained on the publisher's list of The Top Ten Royalty-earning Books for nearly a year. It was published in 2005. See under A. L. Provost at Amazon.com or Barnesandnoble.com.

In addition the interrogator's harmless comment triggered a caveat from the 502 commanding officer when I arrived several months earlier. It was cautionary in nature, and simply stated that if I had any "problems" I was to inform the colonel or one of the other officers discreetly. And even at the young age of twenty-five I was quite capable of reading between the unspoken lines of the base commanding officer. He was of course referring to *mental or emotional problems* brought on as a result of signing a Death Warrant for a North Korean spy once every several months.

Two thoughts wormed their way into my consciousness at the moment. The first, in the form of a question, asked the following:

Was the colonel's open-door policy concerning guidance, offered in the event the job became too mentally or emotionally challenging, offered solely to me because of my youth (I had just turned twenty-five in 1964) or did every new prisoner interrogator receive similar advice? I wondered.

The second thought was that regardless of how mentally and emotionally-challenging the job might become, I was up to the task. I had never been a quitter, not in any endeavor.

I had reached the top of my class at the Defense Language Institute after studying Korean for nearly a year and was at the top of my class after studying Prisoner Interrogation for eight weeks at the U.S. Army Intelligence Center in Baltimore, Maryland. Thus it was my ability to do the job and not my age that landed me the enviable job at the vaunted 502. I silently vowed to meet the challenge of the trust placed in me.

Chapter 22

◇◇◇◇◇

My Fourth Prisoner: The Paratrooper
The Nakasankanghaja Yundae
(The Hidden Paratrooper Regiment)

In an effort to "touch all the bases" in the counterespionage game, following the mad dash to locate the North Koreans' primary goal, i.e., the safehouse, and to apprehend the 3-man espionage team, eventually either Col. Kim or I would walk down the narrow hallway of the I.C. to the file room and retrieve the first of several very thick notebooks.

Back in the I.R. we would place the notebook on the table in front of the colonel and myself, then open the large hardback book to Page 1.

The thick notebook, that we referred to as the *Big Book*, or simply the *Book*, was printed in English. It contained a logical and orderly progression of questions, making the interrogation as comprehensive as possible.

However Col. Kim and I were not tethered to the Big Book; thus it was a *guide* book more than a *cook* book.

One avenue covered extensively in the Big Book related to the enemy *agent's* (not minder's) career in the military. We began with his boot camp and moved him along with the same questions, "And where did you go after that?" (Kutaume udie kasussimnikka?)

From questioning dozens of prisoners we discovered that in arriving at his latest army post the prisoner had followed a similar path, mainly serving in infantry units but occasionally having spent tours in light artillery or heavy mortar batteries. (The Commies were big on mortar batteries.)

In such cases we asked a few detailed questions such as troop strength, ammunition supplies and morale etc., then continued with the next question in the Big Book.

By the time the interrogation team of Kim & Provost had reached its fourth prisoner, each was familiar with the way the other operated. We agreed that if we asked a prisoner a question and the answer contained material that was new to us, instead of showing any surprise we would ask a few innocuous questions, then one of us would announce a coffee break. Leaving the prisoner in the care of one of the Korean M.P.s, we would walk down the hall to the Photography Room to discuss our business in private.

My fourth prisoner was an agent. On the night his 3-man team infiltrated along the South Korean coastline, walking single file they had traveled but a few kilometers when they were ambushed by a ROK Army patrol lying in wait.

Being an agent and therefore unarmed, he threw up his hands immediately. One of the armed minders fired on the ROK Army patrol and was shot dead. The second minder had fled into the thick woods. The agent heard no gunshots, thus had no knowledge of whether the fleeing minder had escaped or had been captured.

The agent carried concealed inside a cloth money belt the requisite $30,000 in U.S. hundreds and $15,000 worth of South Korean *won*. No documents had been found, either on the agent's person or hidden in the woods nearby.

My Prisoner Interrogation Summary following the first day inside the I.C. stated that the prisoner was reasonably cooperative and that he possessed "a military bearing," which was unusual for a North Korean.

Because of this, at the beginning of the second week of interrogation Col. Kim and I decided to track his military bases assignments.

The prisoner went through six weeks of basic infantry training at a base situated twenty kilometers west of the port city of Wonsan.

The answer to our next standard question, "And where did you go after that?" stopped the colonel and me dead in our tracks. It was all we could do to maintain our composure. Following several meaningless, innocuous questions I asked Col. Kim if he needed a coffee break, and minutes later we were standing inside the Photography Room with the door closed.

"Did you hear where his second military base was located?" asked the colonel.

"All I heard him say was that he was posted to a *Nakasankanghaja yundae*, but I'm not familiar with the term," I said, not quite certain why the usually reserved colonel was jumping out of his skin with excitement.

"It's a *parachute regiment*, what the American army calls an Airborne regiment, like the 82nd Airborne or the 101st Airborne." I recall thinking, what in the world have we stumbled onto here? This revelation was big, as in monumental!

"Okay, I'll buy that," I said. "But what am I missing here?"

"What you are missing is the fact that as far as I know – no, as far as anyone in the South Korean Army knows – North Korea does not have any such unit as an Airborne regiment. What do you suggest we do?"

"Let's return to the interrogation room," I said. "I'll let you ask the questions while I write everything down. After about an hour we'll let the prisoner return to his cell. After we go over everything I'll type the Interrogation Summary and take it into Eighth Army to the Twix Center and send it to the Pentagon.

I walked over to the headquarters building and reported our findings to the colonel. While I typed the Summary, labeled *URGENT*, he telephoned the Twix Center and informed the Sergeant on duty to put us at the head of the line when the two American M.P.s and I arrived.

Two hours later I was back at the 502. So as not to alert the prisoner, Col. Kim walked down to the cells. He informed the prisoner that the American had taken ill, and that we would resume the interrogation the following morning.

As with all our teletyped reports to G-2 at the Pentagon, we expected to receive a reply within 3-6 hours. So Col. Kim and I waited around inside the headquarters building, reveling in the importance of our coup, which is exactly what it was. And we both knew we had struck the mother lode.

The much-anticipated call came at 3:30 p.m., but not from G-2 inside the Pentagon. Rather the call was to the commanding officer of the 502, from an official inside the National Security Agency (NSA).

Our colonel was directed to cease all interrogation of the prisoner, and confine the prisoner to his cell for the night. The NSA was flying a two-man interrogation team to Seoul to interrogate the prisoner. This team was expected to arrive at the 502 by noon the following day. The

NSA official also advised our colonel not to discuss the paratrooper revelation with any of the other six interrogators. Fat chance of this advice being heeded! We seven interrogators were a loyal fraternity. The first thing I did was to inform my six comrades.

At 11:45 the following morning a large 4-door black sedan drove up at the gate to the compound. The American M.P. checked the occupants' credentials and waved the car through. The car stopped in front of the I.C. and the two NSA types climbed out, each carrying a small black leather valise.

We seven interrogators were proud of ourselves. We certainly were not envious of the NSA interrogators and actually looked forward to the two men demonstrating their skills. Perhaps we could learn something new.

And we did. An unforgettable experience for certain.

Each small interrogation room had a two-way mirror in the wall facing the narrow I.C. hallway. One could stand in the hall and observe the occupants of the small room but could not be seen by the prisoner. The hallway was narrow but we seven interrogators and Col. Kim weren't about to miss this so we all squeezed together to see the show. The prisoner had already been seated across the table before we arrived at the I.C.

"This is what we had recorded yesterday before the colonel ordered us to cut short the interrogation," I said handing the thin folder to the Caucasian interrogator. He read the several pages, then passed the folder to his African-American partner. Both men appeared to be in their mid-thirties.

The white guy asked us for quiet, then the two entered the interrogation room and sat at the table with their backs to the door.

The scene that played out in that small room and in the crowded hallway was priceless. I'll never forget it as long as I live. None of we seven interrogators ever will.

The black guy spoke first. However we 502 interrogators and Col. Kim didn't understand what he said. We simply looked at one another in puzzlement.

And the befuddled Korean spy just sat at the table appearing quite uneasy. He realized the American was addressing him, yet he certainly didn't understand him. So to avoid incurring the wrath of the two Americans – the ones wearing the spiffy faux-silk suits, – he spoke up, in a respectful tone.

"Nanun tangsinul morogessumnida."

(I don't understand you.)

At this time the white guy, his patience with his partner's questionable translation skills quickly wearing thin, tried out his own Korean on the Korean seated across the table.

The uneasy North Korean spy, his patience with these two also rapidly eroding, spoke up.

"Nanun tangsin-*doe* morugessumnida."

(I don't understand you *either*.)

This awkward impasse was broken by the white guy. Without comment both Americans arose, walked out of the interrogation room and met us in the hallway.

They looked at me and Col. Kim, then the black guy spoke.

"We're not understanding much of what he's saying. What dialect is he speaking?"

"Dialect? There is no dialect. Korean is what we call a *pure* language, same as is English," I said. "A Korean in Pusan, the southernmost port city in South Korea, can be understood by a North Korean living up on the border with China. In other words Korean is Korean is Korean." What followed was likely the fastest exchange of glances ever recorded.

Without further comment the two hotshot NSA *Korean linguists* placed their papers in their valises, walked out the front door of the I.C., climbed into their shiny black sedan and we stood outside the I.C. as the car went through the main gate, then turned left heading in the direction of Kimpo Airport on the way back to Washington, D.C. and the NSA. They didn't appear to be very happy.

And that, as they say in the espionage business, was that, (no) dialect and all.

"Can you imagine the embarrassment this will cause the NSA?" remarked one of the interrogators as we seven plus Col. Kim stood in front of the I.C. wondering what had just happened.

"Colonel Kim, let's walk over to headquarters. We'll tell the colonel what just occurred and I'm sure he'll want us to continue with our interrogation of the prisoner."

Our colonel held mixed feelings concerning the situation. On the one hand the NSA had wasted our time. However at least he would be rid of two government civilians, and in the U.S. Army there was one immutable fact. Civilians loved to pull rank on the military, and all they ever did was get in the way. So none of us was disappointed to see them go.

However before continuing with the interrogation of the prisoner there were two persons who needed to have knowledge of the goings-on.

The CIA Team's Influence

The duo came and went, seemingly with no set schedule. Often they were particularly interested in the aerial photographs that we kept in the Photography Room located at the far end of the narrow hallway in the I.C. Each was a whiz at map-reading and both were quite fluent of course in Korean. Both were always dressed in civilian clothes, were friendly and always available if we had a question for which we did not know the answer.

They worked for the Central Intelligence Agency (CIA). However neither would admit to this, and it would have been rude of us to ask.

Anyway at the time Col. Kim and I walked over to the headquarters building to notify the colonel of the NSA fiasco, we passed the two CIA agents in the hallway. We told them we had an urgent situation, and they invited us into their small office.

"What's the problem Provost?" one of them asked. We showed them the Interrogation Summary we had prepared for the NSA team. It listed the North Korean Army base where the prisoner claimed he had trained as a paratrooper.

"Let's walk back to the Photography Room and take a look at some of the *stock* film of the latest U2 flight," said one of the CIA officers.

In addition to the "special" aerial photography flights, the U2 pilots periodically performed several *flyovers* that covered the entirety of North Korea. Copies of these very detailed photos were stored inside the Photography Room.

Inside the room the CIA agent located the section of the map that included the military base in question. He spread the long photograph out underneath the glass table and slid the large magnifier over the target area.

"I'm not seeing what should be a paratroop training facility," he said after staring at the same area for an inordinate period of time.

"Let me give it a try," said the second agent. He did give it a try, but after several minutes of straining the eyes' ciliary (focusing) muscles, came up short.

"The only possible explanation, that is, if the prisoner is not pulling our leg, is that the base is set up as a normal infantry training base during the day but is converted into a paratroop training facility as soon as the sun goes down late in the day," said the first agent.

"And because the North Koreans probably know we aren't flying the U2 at night, they can set up as many floodlights as they need to make it look like high noon all night long," added the other agent.

"For what little time we've spent with him thus far, he seems to be on the up-and-up with us," I said. "Col. Kim and I are going to continue with this line of questioning, so we should have his answer by the end of the day."

Fifteen minutes later we were back inside our interrogation room. I apologized to the prisoner for having to cut short our *discussion* (it sounded better than *interrogation*) and Col. Kim began by abruptly asking the prisoner, "How late in the day did you begin changing the base over to a nighttime paratroop training facility?"

And he told us.

Everything.

In great detail.

In 1962 when I was the feature writer for the *Stars & Stripes*, the South Korean Army paratroopers held a "drop" of several hundred airborne troops above the giant sandbar that formed an ox-bow near the Han River Bridge south of Seoul.

The paratroopers jumped wearing full battle gear. However the jump master unfortunately was off his calculations, causing the paratroopers to miss the sandbar and more than a dozen of the troops drowned in the deep Han River, pulled under by the weight of their battle gear.

With first-hand knowledge of the South Koran Army paratrooper drowning tragedy from 1962 still stamped indelibly in my memory, I asked the prisoner whether he was aware of any paratrooper "accidents" that might have occurred during training exercises.

Whereupon he related to us an incident he had witnessed personally. On his unit's very first "drop," during daylight hours, ten or more of the 200 paratroopers' parachutes failed to open and the chutists plunged to their deaths. The troops had been forced to fold their own parachutes prior to the "jump."

Col. Kim and I reckoned that the agent paratrooper was so forthcoming concerning the secret base because he did not know that we were unaware of the existence of the base. Certainly we would not let on that we possessed prior knowledge concerning the base. This worked to our advantage.

Our successful interrogation of the agent was a feather in our caps. It made what we did well worth it. Out of curiosity I asked the two CIA agents whether they had been aware of North Korea having paratroopers. They answered in the negative, making our victory even more meaningful.

Col. Kim and I interrogated the paratrooper for longer than two months. He remained cooperative throughout this time, and when I excused myself, strolled down the hallway to collect the Big Book and returned to the room, he seemed to sense the end in sight.

And he was correct, because the Big Book dealt more with the *economy* of North Korea, and the information gleaned from the prisoners supported the general impression we interrogators had that the communist economy was undergoing a rough time.

It was about this time that I became aware of the increase in the number of North Korean prisoners captured and transported to the 502. The paratrooper had been my fourth communist espionage agent interrogated – and executed – in the span of seven months.

And the fate of each of these lost souls, including the fear on the face of each of them as he suddenly came to the realization that the end was in sight, only served to increase the anxiety level of the interrogators themselves. I finally reached the following conclusion.

Shell shock, or at least the effects of the trauma that it produces, is not solely a battlefield phenomenon. Not by the proverbial *long shot*.

Likewise the stress referred to in Post Traumatic Stress Disorder (PTSD) is not confined to battlefield experiences. There was absolutely no doubt in the mind of each of the seven prisoner interrogators that we half dozen plus one would for a long time suffer both the *physical* debility of ulcers as well as the *mental* trauma as evidenced by endless nights of interrupted sleep. These would follow us long after our discharge from the U.S. Army.

Backdrop to the U-2 Incident
The Case for Aerial Photography

Francis Gary Powers was born on August 17, 1929 and died in a civilian helicopter crash on August 1, 1977 at the age of 47.

Powers was an F-84 Thunderjet pilot in January 1956 when he was recruited by the CIA, and in May of that year he began U-2 training in Nevada.

U-2 pilots flew aerial photograph missions mainly over the USSR at heights greater than 70,000 feet. However they were capable of flying special missions nearly anywhere in the world.

In 1956 the United States initiated U-2 flights over the Soviet Union. The Soviet Union possessed radar sensitive enough to pick up the U-2; however it was not until 1960 did the Russians have the expertise to shoot it down.

This occurred on May 1, 1960. Thus the Soviets kept the lid on the fact that they were aware of the aerial reconnaissance flights from 1956 until 1960 because they could ill afford to let the world know that they were aware of America's spying but did not possess the technology to shoot it from the sky.

Powers' U-2 was in the air over Sverdlovsk when it was shot down by an S-75 Dvina (SA-2 Guideline) surface-to-air missile. Upon the missile's impact Powers released the canopy and seat belt. He was captured immediately upon landing by parachute.

On August 19, 1960 Powers was convicted of espionage. He was sentenced to ten years in prison, and was held in Vladimir Central Prison from September 9, 1960 until February 8, 1962, one month after I arrived in South Korea to begin my first tour of duty, on January 3, 1962.

On February 10, 1962 Powers was exchanged for Soviet KGB Colonel Vilyam Fisher, also known as Rudolph Abel. He worked for Lockheed Aircraft as a test pilot from 1962 to 1970, then became a helicopter traffic pilot reporter in Los Angeles.

On August 1, 1977 Powers, along with his cameraman, was killed in a helicopter crash. He died upon impact.

A question often asked was, if as of May 1, 1960 the Soviets – and by virtue of this the North Koreans – were able to shoot down a U-2 aircraft, why didn't the Soviets lend the North Koreans a helping hand?

The general consensus appeared to be that any continuing ill-will between the United States and the Soviet Union simply was not worth the effort. It was a well-known fact that as of the autumn of 1964, upon my return to the 502 following a year at the Defense Language Institute and Prisoner Interrogation at Ft. Holabird, the photos given to us were up-to-date and timely delivered.

The only logical conclusion to be drawn from this was that the Soviets had more important matters on their plate.

Chapter 23

◇◇◇◇◇

Lone Agent – Three-man Team – Lone Agent

Shortly after beginning the interrogation of my first prisoner, and seeking to find the "groove" in my interrogation routine, I came up with what I believed was a brilliant gambit to gain the trust of the prisoner. What's more my scheme involved driving a wedge between the prisoner and his superiors in Pyongyang who had sent him on this suicide mission.

Once I had my plan down pat I approached Col. Kim and we sat aside about thirty minutes during our lunch hour to discuss my plan, that was taken directly from my classes at Ft. Holabird.

When I arrived at the 502, as quietly as was prudent I listened to my fellow interrogators as they discussed their own prisoners. After several months a few patterns began to emerge concerning the relationship between the communist *agents* and their *minders*. The sad basis of this relationship seemed to ring true in every case: No one ever trusted anyone else. Succinctly stated:

The agent did not trust his two minders.

The two minders did not trust their agent.

And the two minders did not trust each other.

The *minders* were supposed to take orders from the agent. The trio was to infiltrate into South Korea, locate the safehouse, carry out the mission (the details of which were known *only* by the agent), then exfiltrate from the coast at night by means of two rubber rafts, to be picked up by a fishing trawler (the details of which were known *only* by the agent).

The prisoner admitted that he had harbored reservations about this plan from the beginning, doubts that surfaced when the two minders never received any map of South Korea and were never taught how to read a map anyway.

By the time of my third prisoner's interrogation I had reached the conclusion that the North Koreans' entire espionage network was predicated on a single premise – distrust.

Love of country and loyalty were absent from the communist ideology, and nowhere was this more evident than in its espionage mission planning. The shocker came however when I came to the realization that the distrust among the agents and minders was *planned*.

And I believed I had discovered the key to the communists' psyche.

In preparation for a spy mission that might require the involvement of more than a single agent, American planners seek out persons who they believe will complement one another, and trust and familiarity are considered essential qualities for success.

The North Korean espionage mission planners however, seek the opposite. In the beginning of the communists' espionage program they likely tried the single agent approach. However the agents realized they could slip away with thousands in American and Korean money, so likely few of these agents were ever heard from again, according to Col. Kim.

Trying the Three-man Team Approach: Distrust

This led to the North Koreans' apparent second approach. They would use three saboteurs, an agent and two minders. Except that to be selected, each of the saboteurs must never had known – or even seen – the other two. They would begin the mission by sowing *distrust* among the three saboteurs, not trust.

The problem with this method became quite evident however, when the South Korean Army reinforced patrols began capturing agents and minders, because it was almost impossible to move three saboteurs about through heavily forested terrain, especially at night.

Because the minders were not given maps nor taught how to use them, the prisoner realized even before the rubber raft carried them to shore that the agent could simply slip away through the woods at night, leaving the minders with no food, no water, no money and no map, and the minders would be at the mercy of South Korean Army patrols and local village police, who because of the sparse population knew everyone in the village and could spot a stranger at more than a hundred yards distance.

At this point in the interrogation the prisoner could not deny the facts as stated above and would confront the stark truth, which was that the minders purposely had been set up to fail by the mission planners back in Pyongyang. Once the agent had arrived safely at the safehouse the two minders became superfluous, literally "excess baggage." To the planners of the mission it was simply too risky to attempt to exfiltrate three communist spies through thick woods just crawling with dozens of trigger-happy South Korean troops.

Once Col. Kim and I had made our point with the minder, it was up to us to link these facts with Col. Kim's assurance that if the prisoner were cooperative and truthful, the colonel enjoyed enough influence with his superiors that he could have the (mandatory) execution set aside in favor of a 20-year prison term.

What made this empty promise quite believable was the stark truth of the first part, because it was an undeniable fact that the Pyongyang planners had set up the mission to fail for the sacrificed minders.

The argument Col. Kim and I made to the uneducated North Korean minder in an effort to "turn" the minder worked more often than not because it was so logical.

For example the reason for the mission planners in Pyongyang allowing the agent and not the minders to carry the food and money never was explained to the minders. However the minders failed to see the logic or fairness in the arrangement, questioning (to themselves of course) what would occur if for any reason they should become separated from the agent and the minders should be left with no food and no money with which to purchase food.

During the course of my sixteen months at the 502 there were numerous instances reported of minders disappearing from the three-member cell, taking some of the money or food with them.

In these cases there was no way to prevent the minders doing this because the agent was purposely unarmed.

I firmly believe that our youth "follows" us. With some rare exceptions our personality at age 30 is nearly the same as it was a decade or two earlier. What psychologists refer to as our "formative" years – teens and early twenties – were just that, so that by the time I entered Berry College I knew my limits when it came to dealing with people.

One of the character traits I acquired during my first year at Oxford Orphanage was a deeply-ingrained sense of empathy – as opposed to sympathy – when I observed a young boy, my age or thereabouts, being mistreated by older boys or heartless cottage counselors and at times even by teachers. Yes, school teachers.

This keen sense of right and wrong was of course still with me the day I arrived at the 502 compound in 1964. I was acutely aware of what was expected of me as a Prisoner of War interrogator, and of the importance of my mission.

However my mindset made a sudden ninety degree turn when I learned that:

The North Korean spies, neither the agents nor the minders, had volunteered for the espionage mission, and the mission planners back in Pyongyang never intended to exfiltrate the hapless minders once the mission had been accomplished.

Thus at the same time the mission planners were demanding loyalty from the *minders* they were purposely keeping from them any maps of North Korea or South Korea while at the same time denying them access to food or money with which to purchase food.

And I would consider myself to be downright disingenuous if I denied that this knowledge affected my interrogations of captured North Korean agents. The only question is the degree to which this in turn affected my own psyche and sense of moral fairness.

Selecting the Minders

After interrogating a number of minders I was able to make a few generalizations as to their qualifications best suited for their mission.

Almost all were drawn from the lowest ranks of the North Korean Army. Thus all had spent time on the rifle and pistol range and had obviously scored high marks with both types of weapons.

All were from small towns or villages, and none had been acquainted with the other members of the 3-man team prior to the beginning of training for the mission. The reason for this practice should be obvious.

Training for the mission lasted generally two months, during which time the minders were forbidden to leave the base or to fraternize with other soldiers. Again an obvious restriction.

From the outset of their training for the mission the minders were given their orders: Protect the espionage agent, who will not be armed. If your 3-man team is discovered by a South Korean Army patrol, do not engage the patrol. Instead, assassinate the unarmed team member, the agent, to prevent his capture. Then commit suicide. Sounded simple enough. That is unless you're the lowly minder.

Aside from this the two minders were instructed to take orders from the agent. The minders were forbidden to handle the map and *were given no instructions to follow* in the event they became separated from the agent.

According to apprehended minders it was at this point they realized that in the eyes of their superiors they were considered to be expendable. And as their superiors denied them access to any kind of map of South Korea, they became prey to any South Korean Army patrol or village policeman, as expendable as a spent .50 cal. brass-jacketed shell on a battlefield.

Assuming that the Americans and South Korean captors would go easier on a lowly, uneducated minder, when captured, the agent did his best to "sell" himself to us as a minder.

However few if any of these feints ever worked for longer than a few minutes. We soon came to the inescapable conclusion that the mission planners back in Pyongyang never intended that the minders return to North Korea. They were totally dependent on the agent for their survival, whereas the agent felt no reciprocal sense of responsibility toward the minders.

First of all the minders never had been taught to read a road map. Not of North Korea. Nor of South Korea. Presented with a road map we could ask the prisoner to trace the "road" from Osan to Taegu. He would choose a line connecting the two towns but fifty percent of the time he would trace his finger along a *railroad track*.

If we asked the minder to point to Seoul he would just stare at the map. He would be completely lost.

Whether out in the woods or inside a safehouse, the agent and the two minders eventually would fall asleep. When the minders awoke hours later they would discover that their lifeline, the agent, was nowhere to be found.

With no money and no way to tell where they were located they became the low-hanging fruit of the espionage tree, easy prey for village policemen or a squad of South Korean soldiers on patrol.

The lot of a North Korean *minder* was not a happy one.

The North Korean mission planners had misjudged the South Koreans however. Recall the facts, that make logical sense.

In 1960 President Syngman Rhee resigned and immediately departed for exile in Hawaii. An interim government never had the confidence of the populace, leaving no one really in charge.

On May 15, 1961 I graduated from Berry College, and on June 30, 1961 I enlisted in the U.S. Army.

On May 16, 1961 General Chung Hee Park took over the South Korean government in a bloodless coup. He established a midnight-to-dawn curfew.

Context was all-important in determining the North Korean mission planners' reason for changing the espionage team's makeup from the single-man to the three-man team.

Following much thought I believed I had hit upon this answer to the problem, because by the time I joined the 502 in the fall of 1964 as the seventh – and youngest – prisoner interrogator, the South Korean Army was scooping up the incoming enemy agents and minders like the latter were pieces of bituminous coal in a wide-mouth flat shovel.

My reasoning – a hunch really – went back to the tyrant president *Syngman Rhee*. Syngman Rhee was an influential South Korean politician who served as the President of South Korea for nearly three terms, from 1948 until his resignation under intense pressure following widespread national protests *in 1960*. Following his resignation he hastily departed South Korea for Honolulu, Hawaii where he died in exile, leaving an economically poor and fractured nation with essentially *no one in charge of the government*. This is the Korea I encountered when I stepped off the thousand-man troopship in Inchon harbor on a freezing, portentous January 3, 1962.

President Rhee's abrupt resignation and sudden departure from South Korea created a power vacuum ripe for communist exploitation. Recall that the Armistice in Korea was signed on July 27, 1953, and economically at least, the country was just as poor seven years later, in 1960.

As far as North Korea was concerned, Kim Il Sung believed South Korea was ripe for the taking, and began flooding the South Korean East Sea with communist saboteurs.

If only it were that simple…

In order to move forward with my theory I needed to determine whether there had been an increase in the number of captured agents and minders following President Rhee's resignation in 1960.

In casual conversation I posed this question to my fellow prisoner interrogator Col. Kim. And his likewise casual answer was in the affirmative. Yes, he said, then added the reason:

The South Korean counterintelligence analysts were convinced the North Koreans increased the number of their spies in order to take advantage of a leader-less country.

On January 3, 1962, seven months after General Park took over the South Korean government, I arrived in Inchon harbor aboard a thousand-man troopship on my way to join the U.S. Fourth Missile Command in Chunchon, the capital of Kangwon Province.

The first night we arrived in Chunchon I observed that every Korean vehicle I saw had its interior lights turned *on*. Because this practice would not be allowed in the United States for obvious reasons, I asked someone the reason for the interior lights being turned on at night.

"This requirement began as soon as General Park took over the government," replied Col. Kim. "Spies could move about the country freely if the interior lights were turned off. So if the interior car lights are turned off, the M.P.s give only one warning. If the driver does not stop, the M.P.s kill all the occupants of the car. There are no excuses or second chances."

This was the South Korea to which I was introduced on January 3, 1962. Believing the South Koreans to be unprepared to defend themselves because of General Park's coup, the communists chose to saturate South Korea with untrained espionage agents.

At about the time I arrived on the scene in January 1962, General Park's military was beginning to have success in capturing members of the three-man North Korean espionage rings. The communists' doubtless desperation in this regard was evidenced by the First Cavalry Division's capture of the Japanese mini-sub containing the body of the drowned North Korean agent in late 1962 while I was still working as the feature writer for the *Stars & Stripes*. The lone-agent and the three-man espionage team were striking out and the Pyongyang planners were becoming desperate.

Hostages?

Renewed success in their search appeared to come with the capture and interrogation of my fifth prisoner. The three-man teams were becoming a disaster, that is until Pyongyang came up with the brilliant (giving credit where credit is due) idea of holding the lone agent's family hostage until the agent completed his mission in South Korea and returned safely to North Korea. In addition the hapless North Korean officer would end up being the proverbial "gift that keeps on giving." The planners could continue sending the officer to South Korea until he was either killed or captured.

I sat back and reviewed the first prisoners Col. Kim and I had interrogated, attempting to discover the reasons the Pyongyang mission planners appeared to be changing tactics. Bear in mind that I was using the data from not only the prisoners Col. Kim and I had interrogated but also data from the interrogations of my six fellow interrogators that I picked up on an almost daily basis during casual conversations. Some thoughts follow.

Now my first and second prisoners had been enlisted men in the North Korean Army. Each had been given but a few weeks of training for the mission, and each had been apprehended by a South Korean Army patrol within a day of coming ashore on the east coast of South Korea.

However my *third* prisoner had been a 35-year-old major in the North Korean Army. My *fifth* prisoner had been an infantry captain in the North Korean Army, thus was an expert in the art of escape and evasion tactics. This fact allowed him to be infiltrated at a greater distance from the safehouse near Sokcho, South Korea.

These facts were pretty much in line with the experiences of other interrogators. Thus beginning shortly after my arrival in the fall of 1964 we were seeing a changeover from the three-man team to the single officer agent.

I passed my theory by our two resident CIA agents as to how, when the single-agent espionage system did not work, the Pyongyang mission planners changed to a just as unworkable system, and when this second (three-man) system also blew up in their faces, someone in Pyongyang came up with the absolutely brilliant scheme to find intelligent and brave North Korean army officers who had parents and other relatives who could be used as hostages to ensure the return of the agent-officer upon completion of the mission.

My theory was bolstered by the apprehension of my fifth prisoner, a North Korean Army infantry captain.

Chapter 24

◇◇◇◇◇

Those Insidious Stomache Pains Begin

The paratrooper came closer than any other captured North Korean agent to having volunteered for the job, because he indeed had volunteered for the army and he, like myself, had confidence in his own abilities.

In addition he was quite insightful, even seeming to be able to pick up on the approximate date of his execution. The information he gave to us, from troop strength to the chronic food shortages, especially in the bitterly cold winter months, was welcomed by the G-2 analysts back in D.C. who, by the way, always wanted more. It's the nature of the army intelligence beast. Yes, thanks, but what else can you do for us today?

As to guessing the date of his execution, more likely the prisoner had learned this from the ROK Army M.P.s who served as guards over the corner of the compound that housed the cells for the prisoners.

The paratrooper was the fourth captured espionage agent I interrogated. And like the three communist spies who took that last ride to The Wall before him he appeared to accept his fate stoically.

Once I had learned firsthand of the mistreatment of the doomed North Korean espionage agents at midnight, I tried my best to put the traumatic events out of my mind.

Couldn't. And I have spent the last half century trying to erase the events of those sixteen months from my memory. Still without success.

Perhaps had I possessed a vent for my spleen, you know like discussing my feelings with a fellow interrogator for example, I might have been able to see my sixteen-month tour of duty at the 502 to the end without my fragile psyche being severely damaged. What the seven of us really needed (but never received) was professional counseling. Lots of it.

Two things constantly nagged at my mind. Probably the same two things that were constantly on the mind of a half-dozen similarly-situated prisoner interrogators at the 502 in 1964-65, to wit:

First I was reminded of the colonel's admonition on my first day back at the 502. If I sensed the job was becoming a problem for me, mentally or emotionally, I was to discreetly notify one of the senior officers in the 502.

Of course then the Eighth U.S. Army shrinks would psychoanalyze me and more likely than not this would be the end of my career as the youngest of seven elite Korean linguists and prisoner interrogators at the vaunted 502.

And knowing myself as well as I did I would brand myself a failure and probably go off the deep end. And this would never do.

And this brought me to the second thing constantly on my mind. Plainly stated, no way in hell would I ever allow any person or any set of circumstances get the better of me. Call me stupid but *failure* has never been an option for me. I would literally die from shame.

So I was stuck with myself, and I just had to make the best of an untenable situation. After all I had done it before. Several times in fact. To me *adversity* has always been just a word in the dictionary, located just before *advert* and just after *adverse*. That's all it is, just a word.

Or rather, I kept telling myself that.

On April 10, 1962, my first day as the new feature writer for the *Stars & Stripes*, I had walked with Jon Powell from the newspaper office to the 502 situated just around the corner, for my first meal in the 502 mess hall.

The first things that caught my eye about the 502 interrogators were the small bottles of a chalky white liquid sitting beside the plate of several of the men. I asked Jon Powell what was the purpose of the bottles of liquid.

"These bottles of the army dispensary's answer to the civilian *Kaopectate*, are used to calm the walls of the stomache," he explained. "These men already have stomache ulcers. It comes with the job."

"And how do we get a diagnosis of ulcers?" I asked.

"Well all I know from the interrogators is that you start getting pains in your stomache area. Not real sharp pains mind you, but enough to keep you awake at night. But there is a quicker, simpler way to diagnose ulcers. If you feel pain in your stomache area just drink a large glass of cold milk. If you have ulcers, the pain will subside when you drink the cold milk."

So when I returned to Korea a year later, following 47 weeks at the Defense Language Institute and eight weeks at the U.S. Army Intelligence Center in Baltimore, Maryland, without informing anyone of my knowledge in this regard I learned as much as possible about the symptoms of beginning ulcers.

I asked several of the interrogators when they first began to notice the stomache pains. The consensus was from four to six months. So at least I knew what to expect.

By the time I filed my Final Interrogation Summary on my fourth prisoner, the paratrooper, and the ROK Army M.P.s came in the middle of the night, loaded him into a crowded paddy wagon for his last ride to an unimposing, nondescript rock wall situated halfway between Seoul and Inchon, I had worked as an interrogator for longer than five months. I still had a year left on my tour. It was still the most exciting time in my young life.

And I was developing chronic, nagging pains in my stomach area. My time had arrived.

Turning Down Reassignment: I Refuse to Quit

We interrogators attached no particular stigma to the affliction of stomache ulcers. The ulcers were not debilitating in the sense that nobody ever lost a day's work because of the condition. With these self-assurances in mind I made an appointment with the Eighth U.S. Army medical dispensary at Yongsan in Seoul.

Following some preliminary tests the physician and I walked into a darkened exam room. He gave me a very large glass filled with a thick substance called *barium* and directed me to stand behind a square-shaped instrument called a *fluoroscope*.

The physician turned on the fluoroscope and directed me to begin drinking the barium. As the barium settled and began coating the inside wall of my stomach he began pressing his fingers onto the outside of the stomach wall through the skin.

"The barium will show me the ulcers inside your stomache by contrast," he said. "It's looking like you definitely have some ulcers. However there are not many of them and the areas of ulceration are not large. We'll give you some medicine that you need to take several times each day. Stay away from the spicy Korean food like they serve in the Chinese restaurants in Seoul."

He added that I should drink a large glass of cold milk sometime during the afternoon.

"Why did I come down with ulcers?" I asked. Dumb question. However as a newspaper reporter I learned never to make assumptions about things of which I had no firsthand knowledge.

"I understand that you are posted out at the 502 Military Intelligence Battalion in Yungdung-po. Is this correct?" he asked.

"Yes I am."

"Then that is your answer. Usually mental stress and worry lead to stomache ulcers. And I can think of nothing that would cause ulcers faster than interrogating communists for so many hours every day. You must be under extreme pressure to produce."

"We are, this is true. But there is another thing that I'm sure makes the situation worse."

"And what is that?" the physician queried expectantly.

"May I speak in confidence?" I asked.

"Confidentiality is mandatory between a physician and his patient, even in the military," he answered. "So what's on your mind?"

I briefly explained to him about the physical abuse suffered by the doomed North Korean espionage agents on the road to Inchon the night of their execution.

"Troops in the 502 have been told that this is a Korean solution to a Korean problem and for us to stay out of it. And they are coming for my fourth prisoner within a night or two."

"So you've experienced *three* of these already?" I sensed a note of incredulity.

"Yes, sir. This will make four executions on the road to Inchon in less than six months."

"And how much longer is your tour of duty supposed to last?"

"Just about a year."

"Provost, I fully understand your dilemma," he said. "If you want to get transferred out of the 502, I'll set up an appointment for you with our medical staff psychiatrist. I feel certain he would recommend a transfer."

"Sir, I really appreciate your advice," I said.

"I just want you to understand the seriousness of your predicament, Provost," he continued. "Ulcers often mask the signs of a deeper psychological problem. In other words your physical discomfort, the ulcers, are the manifestation of a deeper emotional problem. Just give everything a lot of thought. You didn't just wake up one morning with tiny ulcers gnawing at the wall of your stomach. It takes a prolonged period of stress to get to this point."

"Let me think it over sir," I said. "But I asked for this assignment. The army sent me to the Defense Language Institute for a year to study Korean, then to Ft. Holabird, Maryland for eight weeks to study Prisoner Interrogation prior to my coming here. So the army has invested a lot in me, and I am by far the youngest interrogator, at age 25. My leaving would create a problem because they would lose one of the seven interrogators. And there's a matter of pride also in play here."

"I understand," he said. "Just carry on. Take the medicine three times a day. Drink a large glass of cold milk every afternoon and stay away from spicy Korean restaurant food. Good luck to you, and if you ever need me just call."

I never did ask to see the army psychiatrist. But for the next eleven months, until the end of my tour of duty at the 502, I stopped by the Yongsan dispensary once or twice each month just to visit with the physician. Fifteen minutes of mental therapy. Time well spent.

So I joined *The Club*, making it seven guzzlers of the chalky white stomache-coating liquid three times each day plus the large glass of cold milk in mid-afternoon. Following these treatments helped make the ulcers quite manageable.

However I sure did miss that spicy Korean food.

Compensation for the Grief We Suffered?

As discussed earlier the army provided extra compensation for soldiers with a specialized M.O.S. (Military Occupational Skill). This was called *Proficiency Pay*, shortened to *Pro Pay*, and each Pro Pay unit was worth $300.

In addition to my Specialist 5th Class monthly pay of approximately $700, I received one Pro Pay of $300 for being a PW (Prisoner of War) Interrogator and another $300 for being a Korean Linguist. We were paid in cash around the first of each month, so my manila pay envelope held $700 plus $300 plus $300, or $1300.

Pro Pay was similar to, though not the same as *Combat Pay*. It was special pay earned for performing a dangerous duty or in the case of a linguist and prisoner interrogator, a duty for which only a certain kind of soldier has the intelligence, training and education required to attain proficiency.

Not just anyone, regardless of how long he trains, can day in and day out interrogate an enemy agent in the spy's own language and come away with the results attained by the seven interrogators of the 502. And just for the record, we seven weren't just "good," we were "damn good."

There is no doubt in my mind that we all realized our job was taking a toll on our psyche, and looking back on the mental and physical stresses of performing interrogations on North Korean spies six hours daily for months, exacted its toll. I firmly believe that at one time or another each one of us wanted to throw in the towel but realized we would be running away from the fight. Pride was the quality that kept us together and in the end I believe I was a better man because of it. I believe I did my part.

The discovery of the existence of an airborne regiment in the North Korean Army was a feather in my cap from G-2 and a like distinction for Col. Kim from the South Korean Army brass.

Furthermore we could tell that the North Korean Army was unaware of the fact that the Americans were onto the existence of the parachute regiment because the North Koreans never tightened up their procedures of changing the base over to a nighttime parachute training facility.

Chapter 25

◇◇◇◇◇

I Receive a Friendly Warning

There was no rhyme or reason to the order or the identity of the espionage agent to be interrogated by any particular one of the seven interrogators. If I signed the Final Interrogation Summary on a prisoner, like clockwork the oversized paddy wagon drove through the front gate of the 502 compound sometime between midnight and dawn, collected the prisoner and was on its way into the night. The following morning Col. Kim and I would meet at the I.C. at 8:00 a.m., and if there were no prisoner on the Interrogation Schedule we would ask for time off to take care of some personal business. Such requests were always granted.

I surmised that the officers were so lenient concerning time spent away from the interrogation compound was to grant – if requested – a little R&R (Rest and Recreation). Anyway this must have had something to do with it because occasionally for no apparent reason one of the officers would suggest that we borrow a Jeep, drive down to the Yongsan district of Seoul and spend a few hours window shopping at the large Eighth U.S. Army PX (Post Exchange) where one could purchase literally every item that was available in department stores or supermarkets back in the states.

At my visit to the post physician to verify that my chronic stomache pains were the result of ulcers caused by the mental stress associated with the interrogation of captured North Korean espionage agents on a daily basis, I began to quietly observe the other six interrogators, searching for any changes in their personality and demeanor over time.

And I was impressed with the changes of a few of my fellow interrogators. From casual conversation I learned that a particular interrogator was scheduled to end his tour and rotate stateside in four months.

He was approximately thirty-five years old, and I knew him as well as I knew any of our fellow interrogators. He could carry on a decent conversation but was slow at initiating a colloquy, and was for the most part on the "quiet side." He also had begun taking the "white liquid," that I will continue calling by that name although several civilians told me after I mustered out of the army, was likely the drug *Kaopectate*, at the beginning of his fourth month at the 502. And I had been informed upon my arrival at the 502 that 4-5 months was the time the stomache pains began.

Of the six interrogators with me at the 502, a few would speak openly among the others about the prisoner he was presently interrogating. A few others however, did not appear interested in discussing business outside the I.C. This interrogator was one of the latter.

There was an E.M. (Enlisted Men's) club on the small compound, and at times after supper some of the troops (interrogators and support personnel) would meander on over to the club for a beer and some conversation among friends as a means of winding down the day.

One night after supper the interrogator in question and I were seated at a table inside the E.M. club, he nursing a beer and I a Coke. Most of the men had not yet drifted in, so I decided to engage my friend in a little conversation, to "test the waters" so to speak.

"I think you told me before that you were rotating stateside in a few months."

"Yes, it's only four months now."

"Where is your next post?"

"There is none. I'm getting out after these four months. Too much pressure for me."

"I know what you mean by pressure," I said. "I've been taking the white liquid for two months already."

"And from what I hear, you and the rest of us will have ulcers a long time after we are out of the army," he said.

Suddenly I realized what he was referring to. The white liquid would not "cure" the ulcers; the white liquid would take away some of the pain. But the only way to *cure* the ulcers would be to get away from the *cause* of the ulcers, and this meant leaving the 502 and prisoner interrogation behind and entering civilian life.

"Do you recall that on your first day at the 502, one of the officers telling you that if you started feeling depressed, or decided that you did not like your job, to quietly inform one of the officers?"

"Yes, I do recall that conversation."

"Well bear in mind that the officers here at the 502 are constantly observing all seven of us, simply because it is a stressful job. So if one of us suddenly starts bringing up things we object to, like the treatment of the prisoners, they will have that interrogator reassigned. Therefore we don't discuss certain things around here, and they really keep an eye on *you*, Provost."

"On *me?* Why on *me?*" I asked in puzzlement.

"Simply because you are so much younger than the rest of us. So a word to the wise, Provost. Don't have any out-loud conversations with anyone on the compound, especially in the dining hall or here inside the E.M. Club. Do you understand?"

"I understand, beginning right now," I said as two officers entered the club through the front door. A moment later we were discussing the weather and baseball scores.

My friend's warning to me certainly put the quietus on any complaining out loud that I had contemplated. Until the end of my tour.

Chapter 26

◇◇◇◇◇

My Fifth Prisoner: A Change in Tactics?
Family Members as Hostages: An Issue of Trust

Proof that the minders had been sacrificed by the North Korean mission planners in Pyongyang was supplied by a South Korean Army shore patrol unit when it came upon in the deep woods along the craggy East Sea coastline a North Korean espionage agent walking straight into their ambush. Being unarmed and with no chance of escaping, he simply stopped and raised his hands. As of the date of his capture I had been interrogating prisoners at the 502 for nearly eight months, and was well into my third month of medicating myself with the white liquid twice each day.

One of the (many) things that made life at the 502 so interesting was, to employ a trite statement, "every prisoner was different." And this one was. In more ways than one.

The day following my fifth prisoner's arrival he was escorted into the interrogation room by an M.P. and seated across the table facing Col. Kim and myself.

At that first interrogation session, as we went through the preliminary questioning I observed that he was quite cooperative and seemed to be just a smidgen overconfident for my good.

I don't really know why I asked the prisoner the question but something just wasn't kosher. It was as though the prisoner was mocking us. So I interrupted him in mid-sentence with a question:

"You have come to South Korea before today, haven't you?"

Caught off-guard, the answer came as quickly.

"Yes I have. How did you know?"

I simply ignored his question and continued. He was confused, and often this is the best time to pepper the prisoner with questions.

Given a choice the interrogator would rather not deal with an alert, clear-headed prisoner. For obvious reasons.

"How long ago were you here, and what was the purpose of that visit?"

"I was here about eight months ago, and delivered some American money, some South Korean money and some papers to one of our operatives."

"Did you see any of these papers?"

"No, I was told before I left North Korea that the papers were important, but they were secured inside a sealed packet."

"Did anyone come with you this time?"

"No, I came alone; just as on my first mission."

This accounted for the fact he was alone and also unarmed when he was apprehended.

At the time of the prisoner's capture, the South Korean Army patrol recovered the large packets of American and South Korean money and the packet of papers. However the sealed packet of papers contained less than a hundred sheets of cheap North Korean typing paper, with no writing of any kind.

We surmised that the agent was being trained as a courier who could be trusted to deliver sensitive material and cash to agents already ensconced in safehouses inside South Korea. If an agent could be trusted there would be no need to send along two armed minders. And the only purpose in infiltrating teams of agents into South Korea would be to expand the number of espionage cells in the North Korean espionage network.

To me and my fellow interrogators the capture of this agent was significant for another reason. This was my second agent to report that he had been an *officer*, in this case an infantry captain, in the North Korean Army at the time of his being selected to slip into South Korea under cover of darkness. We believed the captain was being trained as a most trusted, loyal courier, charged with delivering the most sensitive orders from the mission planners in Pyongyang.

If this proved to be the case, then how had the mission planners in Pyongyang ensured the captain's loyalty? Especially since "Trust" appeared to be in such short supply in North Korea.

In 1964-65 the South Korean Army patrolled the craggy mountainous coastline generally ten or so miles south of the northernmost South Korean town of Sokcho, because it was a known fact that the longer an agent and his minders were far from their destination, the greater the chance of being spotted by a South Korean Army patrol. However upon questioning, the captain reported that he had been dropped off by a rubber raft nearly *fifteen* miles away. The reasoning for this he claimed, was that as an infantry captain he had been taught how to elude the South Korean Army patrols.

During this time period 1964-65 the South Korean Army patrols enjoyed a great deal of success in tracking and either killing or apprehending spies from the north. And as soon as the North Koreans increased the number of agents being infiltrated into South Korea in order to fill the void created by the loss of agents, the South Korean Army stepped up its number of patrols, according to Col. Kim. In this race for attrition the South Korean Army was definitely coming out ahead.

The prisoner confirmed some of our suspicions in explaining his mission.

"Were you aware that the packet you brought with you contained only blank sheets of paper?" asked Col. Kim.

"No, I did not know that," responded the prisoner.

"Do you know the reason for this?"

"North Koreans never trust one another," said the prisoner. "I believe they were testing my loyalty before they allowed me to carry any valuable material. But they had no reason to question my loyalty."

And just why was this, I wondered.

It was quite possible the communist planners had miscalculated the degree of risk likely involved in sending a sole agent on these missions. The captain appeared resigned to his fate, and even more important, to the fate of his *family*. He answered our questions openly, the veracity of his answers being confirmed quite easily by the use of U2 aerial photographs. Col. Kim and I reasoned that the prisoner's cooperation was his final revenge for the treatment he and his family had endured at the hands of the mission planners in Pyongyang.

"Why is this?" asked Col. Kim.

"Because my family, including my mother, my father and my younger brother, live in a small village near Pyongyang. If I do not return from this mission the government will send my family to a work farm, which is the same as a prison. They'll die there."

"Did you volunteer for this mission?" asked Col. Kim, knowing what the answer would be.

"No, In North Korea nobody ever asks you to volunteer for anything. They just point a finger and you follow them."

Assuring the Enemy Agent's Loyalty

The capture of the North Korean officer was significant for a number of reasons. This was the first time Col. Kim and I had interrogated an officer who had admitted to having *come alone*. Upon inquiry Col. Kim confirmed this. And to the best of my knowledge none of my fellow interrogators had ever interrogated an agent who acted alone. Up to this point anyway.

However this reasoning possessed merit. It certainly would create less attention using a single agent who was an expert in cover and concealment, as opposed to three agents stumbling around through miles of thick forest at night.

Thus the Pyongyang mission planners assured the loyalty of the espionage agent simply by holding his family hostage. Col. Kim and I agreed that the communists would continue to use the courier until the day he was captured or killed by a south Korean Army patrol. Furthermore because the agent's family would have no way to confirm that the officer was dead, the man's family likely would still end up in a work camp. From the outset the hapless North Korean officer must have known the situation would never be resolved in his favor.

For the communists their loss of an officer was definitely a gain for us. He spoke freely and did not appear evasive in answering our questions.

The captain realized he never again would see his family and that in all likelihood the family members would die of starvation in a work camp the following winter.

In my next Interrogation Summary I added our conversation with the captain and detailed my thoughts concerning my belief that the North Koreans were experimenting with a single-agent method of espionage.

My next question concerned whether this subtle change in the communists' makeup of their 3-man infiltration system in favor of the single-agent system had been experienced by any of the other six 502 interrogators. Three of these six had indeed encountered this change in tactics by the Pyongyang planners. I added this information to my next Interrogation Summary. The analysts at G-2 in the Pentagon would be pleased with this news and with our analysis.

The captain's interrogation, that could best be described was a *debriefing* given the amount of valuable information he divulged freely, lasted a little longer than two months. On the final day, as I walked out the door of the interrogation room, without comment I paused and shook hands with the captain. Neither of us spoke.

I found it difficult to get to sleep that night; the captain's utter loss of self and family being likely his final thoughts as he stood in front of a rock wall out in a field halfway between Seoul and Inchon, awaiting the end.

Doubts Concerning the Three-man Espionage Team

Shortly after interrogating my third prisoner I had begun to question the efficacy of the communists' employment of the 3-man espionage team. One day I paused mentally and wondered why the communist mission planners had settled on this very cumbersome method of spying. But until I could figure out on my own the possible whys and wherefores, I didn't want to make a fool of myself by broaching my concerns to my fellow interrogators.

So I donned my thinking cap and tried to approach the problem in a logical manner.

And it was something the fifth prisoner said that whetted my interest. My first question:

Why did the planners in Pyongyang settle on the 3-man team initially? This answer was supplied by several of the agents and minders I had interrogated previously. The answer? Because there was no way the mission planners could *Trust* just a single agent. And this had presented a major roadblock in achieving success in their method of infiltrating agents into South Korea.

Then I recalled that when I had questioned the captured agents and minders about their family, none had expressed fears concerning the safety of family members.

That is until the fifth agent. Inserting my sluggish mind into the pencil sharpener labeled "Reason," I gave the handle about twenty rapid turns and donned my thinking cap. After giving the problem much thought I developed my theory of the communists' change in tactics from the 3-man team to the lone agent method of espionage. For answers I consulted the two resident CIA agents.

"Provost, you're expressing the same concerns as are several of your associates. And this is what we have come up with so far," one of the CIA agents said. His paraphrased explanation follows.

In order to establish a network of communist cells in South Korea, the mission planners must have some way to funnel money and instructions into the country. But this creates a problem. Unless there is a way to exfiltrate these agents out of South Korea along the east coast, it is impossible to determine whether or not the mission was successful.

Because initially the reliability of the one-agent method was highly questionable, this forced the Pyongyang planners to try other methods.

"Provost, do you recall the Japanese mini sub disaster that occurred when you were with the *Stars & Stripes* a year or so ago?"

"Yes I do. What a dumb idea that was."

"And do you recall them trying that same stunt here recently, with the same results?"

"Yes, I do." This indeed had occurred.

"Trying it the first time was a desperation measure. Repeating it a year or so later only showed how really desperate they were."

It all boiled down to *trust*, said the CIA agent. There is not a single North Korean who asked to become a spy. This forced the mission planners to set up the 3-man system, just so the espionage agents could keep an eye on one another. And this distrust of each other is what leads the 3-man teams to fall apart. It simply doesn't work.

In addition the fact that the planners intentionally ensured that the three members of the team had never met until a few weeks before the mission, also worked against the success of the mission because the planners sowed distrust among the three from the outset.

During the last eight months of my 16-month tour the number of North Korean agents captured each month decreased slightly. Possibly two thirds of those captured were *lone agents*, and the majority of those lone agents had been drawn from the officer ranks of the North Korean Army. Reports from my fellow interrogators indicated that nearly all of the lone agents had relatives in North Korea, ensuring as best the communists could the enforced loyalty of the agent.

In effect the mission planners replaced three *amateur* agents with one *professional* agent, a mature North Korean Army infantry officer, adept at escape-and-evasion tactics.

This was definitely a step in the right direction. However there remained one lingering problem: How do the brilliant mission planners secure the loyalty of this lone agent? The answer was obvious:

Simply by holding the agent's family members hostage, as had been done with my fifth prisoner, the North Korean Army infantry officer.

Chapter 27

◇◇◇◇◇

My Sixth Prisoner:
A Liar's Trip to Yongsan: The Polygraph

Occasionally a prisoner would demonstrate a rare degree of intelligence as well as the knowledge of his mission, such that we afforded him some latitude in the form of tolerating his behavior. In other words we would ignore a degree of evasiveness in hopes we would not be required to call the Korean army colonel to take him away at midnight for an "attitude adjustment," South Korean Army style.

Trouble was, sometimes the prisoner would catch on to the fact he was getting special consideration and would begin fabricating stories in an attempt to confuse and mislead us. This created a dilemma of sorts, as follows.

We could contact the Korean Army and inform them that a certain prisoner was lying to us or else was giving us conflicting stories. The paddy wagon would pull up in front of the prisoner's Quonset-hut cell that same night, collect the frightened prisoner and drive off into the darkness of the narrow Seoul-Inchon road.

The South Korean Army's treatment of the prisoner generally brought instant results. The prisoner usually began talking the following day. Trouble was we couldn't shut him up. It's as though someone had wound up the Energizer Bunny and turned him loose, and suddenly we were inundated with TMI – Too Much Information. And most of it questionable. Telling us what he thought we wanted to hear.

And this is the point at which an interrogator brought up the idea of using the polygraph in similar situations. I wish the idea had been mine but sadly I cannot take credit for it. And anyway, this was before my time.

However Col. Kim had had several years' experience in matching wits with enemy agents. I noticed from the beginning of our interrogation that the colonel had very little patience with the prisoner, because the prisoner appeared to change his mind concerning seemingly trivial parts of his story.

At 4:00 p.m. on the Friday ending our second week of interrogation, the South Korean M.P. guard escorted the prisoner back to his cell for the weekend, while the colonel and I prepared to type our interrogation summary for the day.

As mentioned earlier we had been instructed to include with each summary a statement as to whether we believed the prisoner was being truthful with his answers to our questions. However Col. Kim appeared to be in a pensive mood when we took our seats in the typing room at company headquarters.

"Something bothering you, colonel?" I asked. Often prisoners would give us a hard time for the first several days of their interrogation, because they were downright scared out of their wits at having been captured by the South Korean Army.

However they generally settled down once they knew more or less the interrogation routine. But following a week of interrogation, this prisoner appeared to be stuck in a combative stance, more like a petulant child than a North Korean spy.

"Yes Provost, what's bothering me is that the prisoner has been feeding us a string of lies, enough that I believe we should take him for a ride to Yongsan."

"Do you mean we should call the Korean Army to take him away for the night to do whatever they do to stop his lying?" I asked.

"Not exactly," explained the colonel. "This particular prisoner is a captain in the North Korean Army. He appears to know a lot, and might respond in a negative way to force or threats of force, although a nighttime ride in a paddy wagon is still an option."

"So what do you suggest?"

"When it has to do with prisoner interrogation you, Provost, control what happens. I believe we should set up an interview with the polygraph examiner, whose office is located at Eighth U.S. Army Headquarters on the Yongsan compound in Seoul."

"Who questions the prisoner during the test?"

"Not us," said the colonel. "There are Korean interrogators at Yongsan who perform the actual polygraph exam. We'll go through our interrogation summaries and pull out the questions on which we believe the prisoner has lied. Then the Yongsan interrogator asks the prisoner these questions again."

"Does the polygraph operator tell the prisoner he thinks the prisoner is lying, if this happens to be the case?"

"No, this will be our job once we get him back to the 502. My feeling is that he is lying more often than he is being truthful."

I felt as though this was Col. Kim's show because he had been at this game for several years when he and I first met. The questions we turned in to the Korean interrogator – polygraph operator at Yongsan included questions we had previously asked plus any other questions we intended to ask as part of our interrogation. Col. Kim submitted eleven questions for me and twenty-seven questions for himself.

At 8:00 a.m. on the day of the polygraph examination the M.P. guard marched the prisoner to the I.C., but instead of escorting him into the building he placed the surprised North Korean Army captain inside the paddy wagon parked on the street.

Col. Kim and I were standing nearby and observed the expression on the face of the prisoner as he was led not toward the I.C. but toward the cramped, foreboding paddy wagon. To this day I feel that the prisoner believed he was being escorted to the site of his execution.

On the way to Yongsan Col. Kim and I followed in another Jeep, with the colonel holding the valise that contained the list of questions. Inside the Polygraph Room Col. Kim handed the valise to the interrogator, who withdrew the papers, scanned the questions briefly, then placed the papers face-down on the table.

"They are going to bring the prisoner in and sit him at the table facing me," he said. "You can observe as they hook him up to the equipment, through the one-way glass," explained the polygraph operator.

The operator explained that the polygraph examination was not based on an exact science because there are too many variables, one of which was the emotional state of the subject being tested.

"So what I say to you is that *to the best of my knowledge* the prisoner is – or is not – telling the truth, in response to a particular question. That's all I can say."

Col. Kim and I stood looking though the glass window out of sight of the prisoner, while the interrogator completed his preparations.

The interrogator's only comment to the prisoner was to the effect that he was going to ask the prisoner some questions. That's all. Not once did he admonish the prisoner to be truthful because, he said, a polygraph examination does not allow for conversations, extraneous words, phrases or comments.

We had prepared 38 questions for the polygraph operator, 11 from me and 27 from Col. Kim. Not rushing the prisoner, the test took about an hour and fifteen minutes. I believe the prisoner caught on to what was happening on about Question No. 5.

When we returned to the 502 the prisoner was escorted straightaway to our interrogation room. Col. Kim and I sat across the table, and the colonel placed his valise on the table, withdrew the test papers and turned them to where the prisoner could read them.

Col. Kim called the prisoner's attention to one of the questions. Pointing to the question, Col. Kim accused him of lying. Immediately the excuses spewed from the liar's mouth. I was nervous. I didn't understand the question. The examiner was speaking too fast. And on and on.

But Col. Kim would have none of it. He stated his case in a calm, matter of fact tone.

"We told you on the first day that if you answered our questions truthfully, we could assure you that you would spend the next twenty-years in prison, but you would not be executed. And this is how you repay our kindness? Well?"

At this the lying North Korean agent saw his life coming to a crossroads, because the questions the examiner checked had been those in which he had lied. With no way out he threw himself on Col. Kim's mercy.

"I made a mistake colonel," he began, his voice somewhat less confident than the day before.

"I would have to agree with you," responded Col. Kim. "You have wasted our time is what you have done."

"Can I start over? I will answer all your questions truthfully. It was my mistake. It will not happen again."

"We will continue with our questions," said Col. Kim. "However we will also take you to be tested every week. If you lie to us even one more time, we will be unable to save you from your execution."

The captain turned out to be one of the better educated of all the North Korean agents whom we interrogated. However the rash of lies he told us, leading to the polygraph examination, never did sit well with Col. Kim. Or with myself for that matter.

However we did send him to Yongsan once each week during the two months he was our "guest" at the 502, and to the best of my knowledge he never lied to us again.

However before the end of my tour, what we interrogators came to refer to as simply the "record," occurred. We never did understand how the interrogator's prisoner pulled it off, however before the smoke had cleared, he had managed to change his name *nine* times. Finally disgusted at the insult, the American interrogator and his South Korean Army counterpart placed the North Korean agent's name on the midnight paddy wagon list. In only one night it ended all the enemy agent's foolishness. Sang like a communist bird, he did. More fun and games at the 502. Never a dull moment.

Observations, Generalizations and Conclusions At the End of My Tour at the 502

There is no doubt in my mind that at least for the period beginning January 3, 1962, when I took my first tentative steps off the thousand-man deathship in Inchon harbor, and ending on November 4, 1965, when I boarded the huge four-engine propeller-driven passenger plane at Kimpo Airport for my return to the states, that at the end of this nearly five-year period, I knew *more than* any other American about South Korea, and *as much* about communist North Korea as did any other American. Probably more.

My observations of the Two Koreas alone likely would occupy several hundred pages, and every one of these stories would be just as interesting as I hope you have found the enclosed accounts to be. To recount just a few of the more memorable situations:

Based on prisoner interrogations, North Korea was a dirt-poor country whose communist government could not adequately feed and clothe its population. Malnutrition was the menu for the day, and statistics showed that only twenty percent of the land would sustain agriculture. South Korean winters were harsh; *North Korean* winters were brutal, for weeks on end.

There is a truism floating around in the American law enforcement ether that holds that what befalls most crooks is not the brilliance of law enforcement but rather the stupidity of the criminals. Stands to reason.

A similar rule holds for the North Korean communist infiltration of South Korea. Their system was poorly planned and singularly amateurish. The South Korean Army shore patrols were efficient and aggressive, scooping up the ill-trained communist infiltrators almost as soon as they came ashore. Business was always good at the 502.

The U.S. Army's prisoner interrogation system was top-notch and quite professional. We helped one another, sharing our personal experiences and interrogation techniques. The instruction we received at both the Defense Language Institute and the U.S. Army Intelligence Center was first-rate and definitely allowed us to "hit the ground running" when we arrived at the 502.

I had applied myself diligently at both these schools and realized that because I was by far the youngest prisoner interrogator at the 502, likely my conduct at the interrogation center would remain under scrutiny until I had *proven* myself, in the eyes of both the officers and my fellow interrogators.

The biggest compliment I received was when after I began the interrogation of my third prisoner, the other interrogators started asking my opinion on interrogation techniques. At that point I realized I had been accepted among my peers. It meant a lot.

Thus I am pleased to report that apparently I passed muster, because in my exit interview with our commanding officer he praised me for my interrogation skills and was sincere when he asked me to reconsider my decision to end my army career at the end of my tour of duty at the 502.

Thus living conditions during the time I spent in South Korea (January 1962 – November 1965) were woefully inadequate for both populations. I would like to touch briefly on several of these disheartening examples that I witnessed first-hand when I began working at the *Stars & Stripes*.

The Plight of Vagrants and Streetwalkers

Signs of this abject poverty were clearly evident on the streets of Seoul. I'll mention just a few cases. In early April, 1962 I began working as the feature writer for the *Stars & Stripes*. The newspaper offices and living quarters were located in a two-story converted red brick warehouse in Yungdung-po, a residential district south of the Han River. As the feature writer I had assigned to me on a permanent basis, a Jeep. I had freedom to travel alone the entire country, and I could stop by any military post to eat, sleep, then gas up my trusty Jeep and be on my way. What a life!

In writing my stories I often left early in the morning and returned late at night. And to reach most of my destinations, that were usually *north* of Seoul, I had to cross the Han River Bridge and pass by the Seoul Central Train Station near the center of the city.

On the sloped northern bank of the Han River as I crossed the bridge at daybreak on that first morning, I looked off to my left front and right front to observe some of the most beautiful teenage girls and young women I had ever seen, slowly emerge from literally dozens of what could best be described as cardboard hovels, and make their way toward Seoul along streets and dirt sidewalks.

The scene was singularly surreal, and I made a mental note to ask the other reporters about it upon my return to the newspaper later in the day.

However I encountered several delays along the way to and from my story, such that it was past midnight when I approached the Seoul Central Station heading south. Because an enforced curfew existed during those turbulent times, the streets around the rail station were clogged with vehicles trying to get to their destination before their chariots were transformed into pumpkins.

As I drove slowly past the train station suddenly I heard cries of pain amid yells of insult. The former emanated from the ragged pedestrians huddled as close to the station as possible, while the latter proved to be a dozen or more Seoul policemen swinging black wooden truncheons in an effort to dislodge the vagrants and send them on their way. So now I would be seeking explanations to two phenomena, which I mentioned at breakfast the following morning. The two explanations were indeed eye-openers. A veritable clash of cultures before my very eyes!

The early-morning exodus from the cardboard shanties, explained Jon Powell, were young women on the way to cruise the streets of Seoul to sell their bodies to G.I.s inside the bars.

"That's a lot of beautiful girls," I said. "Don't they have regular jobs?"

"That's the crux of the problem, in a nutshell," responded Powell. "Simply stated, there are no jobs. The economy is shot to hell, and the South Korean government is corrupt. Unless someone takes over and establishes order, this situation will never improve."

The second problem – the vagrants at the train station – proved to be tied to the first, the young female streetwalkers. The vagrants' refusal to leave the train station at midnight was because they had no homes. Therefore when they were rousted from the train station, they were still violating the curfew unless they were *inside a building*. The Seoul police however could live with the vagrants walking the streets. These streets just could not be in downtown Seoul.

"Welcome to the real world, Provost," said Jon Powell. I realized I had a lot to learn.

Desperate Times Call for Desperate Measures
No, I Don't Want her.
What Would I Do With Her?

A week or so after observing beautiful young women and girls emerging from the north bank of the Han River and that same night witnessing the Seoul police's assault on the vagrants milling about the Seoul Central Train Station, I left the *Stars & Stripes* building heading north to write a story on a 155mm Howitzer unit located in the First Cavalry Division near Uijongbu in the DMZ. Having trained on the smaller, much shorter-range 105mm (Range seven miles tops) while stationed at Ft. Sill, Oklahoma, I was quite eager to see the 155mm version of the "big gun" in operation.

The closer one came to the DMZ, the more the *paved* roads became the norm. I do recall that a light rain was falling at the time so I slowed quite a bit when I observed several adults and children walking on the *right* side of the road and about twenty or so yards to my front.

As I closed the distance between myself and the pedestrians to about ten feet, suddenly a teenage girl entered the road from my *left* and yelled. This caught my attention and I glanced toward her. I recalled thinking – just where in the hell did you come from, little girl?

In that brief one-second interval between the time I heard the girl to my left yell and I turned my head in her direction I heard a *ker-THUNK* sound of something hit metal really hard. When I stopped my Jeep and looked to my right I observed one of the young women sprawled out on the road. Seeing her in that position, my first thought was that if I had hit the girl with my Jeep, it certainly had not knocked her down (and it appeared – out) because my Jeep had barely been moving when the girl collided with the vehicle. From the very beginning I smelled a shakedown.

I quickly knelt down beside the fallen girl. Her breathing appeared normal. However if she were attempting to convince me she was unconscious, she wasn't exactly slated to win an Academy Award for her performance.

True, she appeared to be unconscious. However her brow definitely was furrowed, and her eyelids were closed tightly. Just as I suspected, I was being "set up." The road traffic from Seoul to Uijongbu was fairly heavy, so I flagged down the first Jeep to come down the road.

I explained to the driver what had occurred and the reasons I suspected a shakedown. He got on his telephone and ten minutes later a Jeep carrying two M.P.s arrived on the scene. I followed in my Jeep to the dispensary a few miles away.

The medics examined the girl, who by some miracle had opened her eyes as soon as the medics placed her on the guerney at the site of the so-called "accident." The medics found no signs of trauma anywhere on her body. I explained to them what I believed had occurred.

The M.P.s conferred with the medics and we walked out to the lobby of the dispensary. The older of the M.P.s spoke.

"Provost, get back into your vehicle and continue on your way. These poor Korean families have no income or way to earn a living, so it's hard to fault the girl. What they would like is for you to take care of her and her family." Then turning serious, he asked, "You don't need a girlfriend, do you? She certainly is a beauty."

And he was dead serious.

"No, sergeant, I don't want her." Then hesitating I asked after a beat, "What would *I* do with her?"

"Just thought I'd ask," he replied smiling. "You never can tell."

Upon my return from writing the article about the 155mm Howitzer company I told my story to the other guys at the newspaper.

"Get accustomed to it Provost," said Sergeant Kelsey. "Do you recall how loud was the sound when your Jeep struck her?"

"Yes, I did notice the loud sound."

"Well that was the sound of her fist striking the hood of your Jeep, and was done to convince you that you had caused a serious collision. Forget it Provost. It'll happen again."

And it did. At least a half dozen times during the following year. The reason I appeared to be ideal for a shakedown was because I was traveling *alone*. In other words there was no one to back up my version of the story, i.e., that I did not cause the accident. If there existed no visible signs of trauma, the M.P.s weren't about to waste their time pursuing the matter.

The War I Missed – And Was Glad of It

I never have minded taking chances. That is, as long as I believe I stand a pretty good chance of surviving whatever it is I'm risking. A little wordy there; however I believe you get my drift. So here are the facts. It's an interesting story.

After completing Basic Infantry Training at Ft. Jackson, South Carolina in September 1961 and Advanced Artillery Training at Ft. Sill, Oklahoma in late November 1961, my company commander at

Ft. Sill, Captain John Corning, told me to hang around until the next Officer Candidate School (OCS) class opened up.

Following several weeks of slurping sodas and trying out every combination of ice cream known to man, one morning Captain Corning asked me to stop by his office "to sign some papers," he said.

An hour later I knocked on his office door and he welcomed me in. I pulled up a chair and sat across from him at his desk. He reached into the wooden tray resting on the corner of the desk and withdrew several typed pages. There were blank spaces at the bottom of each page. Like for example, spaces for signatures maybe?

The captain explained the situation briefly, an explanation I had not received up until then. I had no explanation for this gross oversight on the army's part, but the situation was to become moot anyway.

I had signed up for the standard three-year tour when I enlisted on June 30, 1961. However the army's rule was that in order for an OCS candidate to attend OCS, there had to be at least three years *remaining* on his enlistment at the time he graduated from OCS.

"So how do we correct this oversight?" I asked although I was certain I knew the answer.

"The only way is for you to sign up for an additional three-year tour," he said.

However six years in the army simply was not in the cards – at least not those in my deck of shiny plastics anyway.

Almost without hesitation I asked, "So what are my options, sir?"

He pointed to the papers in the wooden tray. "If you sign this paper, you will not go to OCS. You'll just go back into the *pool*. Within a month you'll be assigned to your next post. Nobody knows where this will be because these assignments are made at the Pentagon in Washington, D.C."

I thanked the captain for his help, and wished him well.

"I'm getting out of the army Provost, following the tour I'm presently on." he said.

"Why so, sir?" I asked.

"Well the war in Vietnam is just starting to get really nasty, and I want no part of it," he replied. "You're a good guy Provost. I hope for your sake that you don't get sent over there."

And this was the start of the *Big Worry*. The situation began with *Bad*, slipped into the gear called W*orse* and seemed to be heading inexorably at breakneck speed toward *Worst*.

At that point my newspaper keyword became *Vietnam*. I read every newspaper I could get my hands on, eagerly searching for this Vietnam. And the captain had (unfortunately) been spot-on in his assessment of the situation. It was November 1961. My meticulous research using back issues of the *San Francisco Chronicle* and *Newsweek, Time* and a few other monthly magazines published in late 1960 and early 1961 produced the following worrisome information.

I had graduated from Berry College on May 15, 1961. On May 11, 1961, just four days before my graduation, President John F. Kennedy ordered 400 Special Forces troops to South Vietnam and authorized covert military operations. The U.S. Army referred to these elite troops as *advisors*. Yeah, you bet! Advisors my eye!

On November 22, 1961 President Kennedy authorized a major escalation of American involvement in South Vietnam, including military helicopters. On the date of this announcement I received the cautionary warnings from the captain, and I began to worry about my future.

A few days later my orders came to company headquarters, and Captain Corning called me into his office. He read the orders, smiled and we shook hands. The orders directed me to travel immediately by passenger train from Ft. Sill, Oklahoma to Oakland, California, then travel by troopship from San Francisco to South Korea, and from there by Korean passenger train to join the U.S. Fourth Missile Command at Camp Page in Chunchon, capital of Kangwon Province, way the hell up in the boondocks.

My concerns were well-founded, as I could read the portentous word *escalation* in the events of the following year, 1962. By December 31, 1961, there were approximately 900 American military personnel in South Vietnam. Five American soldiers had already been killed in combat.

A year later, on December 31, 1962 there were 3,200 U.S. military personnel in South Vietnam, and the death toll for 1962 had risen to 16.

What continued to cause a chill running up and down my spine for longer than a year following my arrival in Korea was the knowledge that following my decision to opt out of Officer Candidate School in November 1961, the army could just as easily have ordered me to Vietnam as it had to South Korea.

And I to this day quite vividly view in my Single Lens Reflex the image from the front page of the *Stars & Stripes* that depicted Gen. William Westmoreland addressing his troops following a battle, with the seventeen dead U.S. soldiers filling the black body bags laid out in two rows before him. Bone-chilling view it was. Certainly a memory to last a lifetime.

Seemed as though once the Vietnam War got into my system, it held on for as long as it could. When a planeload of G.I.s arrived at the air base north of San Francisco, scheduled to be processed out of the army at the end of their tour, the group traveled by bus to the Oakland Processing Center. I was in this group of about 150, eager to muster out of the service and get on with our lives. Processing was scheduled to take about two days.

We grabbed our duffel bags from off the bus and walked into a large room inside the processing center, and took our seats. A colonel addressed the group. He was not smiling.

"Men, we are scheduled to begin our two-day processing tomorrow morning. However there is an airplane coming in tonight from Vietnam. Because these men are coming from a war zone, they are automatically given priority in being processed out of the army. We hope you understand."

Well, the plane from Vietnam landed that night, and we had to hang around the processing center for three days before beginning our processing, that lasted for another two days. There was an amount of grumbling from our group of 150, but most of us just took the delay in stride and eventually I made it home.

My *Adventure* was over, and I was happy just to get on with my civilian life. However at times when I find myself in a nostalgic fog, I think of what might have been. And shudder.

Epilogue

End of the Adventure

Eventually it came time to leave Korea, to get off that four year, four month and four day detour and back on to the interstate called *LIFE*, to part company with the United States Army and put more than a little distance between myself and the infamous 502. Little did I know it then, but trading my Army Green for civvies would take an adjustment similar to the one I had made going the other way several years earlier. Egads! What a rollercoaster of a ride that had been.

Destiny is defined as "the seemingly inevitable or necessary succession of events; what will necessarily happen to a particular person."

When applied to the facts of my life, this book could well have been titled *My Destiny*, because these events appeared to fall into place, time-wise, as though they were pieces of an interlocking jigsaw puzzle.

My four and a half year adventure stresses the need to be prepared for life's numerous possibilities, to position oneself to grab the proverbial brass ring as the world whistles by, with no second chances in sight.

My DD Form 214 indicates that I served my country honorably for the four years, four months and four days of my enlistment. However even as three of my prisoner interrogator friends accompanied me on my final drive to Kimpo Airport on that chilly November 4, 1965 mid-morning, I sensed that the 16-month experience and my psyche would remain tethered to one another for many years, if not forever.

On the morning of my final departure from Korea, as the huge four-engine passenger plane thundered down the runway at Kimpo Airport, I uttered a final prayer – foolish mortal, I – that somehow I might be able to escape the notorious 502 and the midnight screams of the doomed communist espionage agents on the way to their execution at The Wall.

Fifty odd years later I have yet to fully succeed in this endeavor. Thus to revert to the vernacular, I suppose I'm stuck with myself.

On the hour-long drive to the airport the four of us traded stateside hometown addresses, promising to stay in touch. Several weeks later I received a letter in the mail. My fellow interrogator asked whether I recalled a specific prisoner by name.

As much as I liked and respected my friend, I never answered his letter. Fifty years later I still believe I did the right thing. For my sanity if for no other reason. I never answered any of the half-dozen or so letters I received. I only hope my friends understood and forgave me.

Truth be told the pangs of nostalgia and loss hit me in the gut a few weeks prior to my Honorable Discharge, and I realized just how much the friendship, camaraderie and service to country had meant to me. Still does, after more than half a century.

Please feel free to quote me in this regard, but millions of American veterans will vouch for the fact that once an American puts on a U.S. Army uniform, he will never again be the same person he was prior to "joining up." To the contrary, he will be a better person for the experience.

I have always been proud of my years wearing the Army Green, and it is possible I might have had a few misgivings about ending my time as the youngest *Stars & Stripes* reporter and sole feature writer and the youngest Prisoner of War interrogator at the 502, half a century ago.

But only a few. Sometimes a man just has to move on, to discover what's waiting for him on the far side of that expansive, lush-green pasture philosophers call *life*. As one famous writer mused, life is not a destination but a journey. I can see his point.

Again, I would not trade the years I served in the U.S. Army for all the tea in China. I am happy to have had the experience, and if asked, I would do it all over again in a heartbeat.

Upon reflection many years after what today I refer to as *My Grand Adventure* at times and *My Unbelievable Experience* at others, my busy life in my post-Korea era has rescued me from being a slave to nostalgia.

Thus it has finally come time to sign off, so I'll end where I began this topsy-turvey tale. Recall the ephemeral experience and the Tar Baby experience? What have I learned from my four year, four month and four days during which my life was controlled by the U.S. Army?

I learned to be proud of America's military. I learned that the army runs on the merit system and that age has nothing to do with it. I was the youngest reporter at the *Stars & Stripes*. Yet I was the feature writer, was entrusted to cover the meetings of the Military Armistice Commission at Panmunjom, and was the only reporter who held a Top Secret Security Clearance.

Likewise I was far and away the youngest Prisoner Interrogator at the 502, having just turned twenty-five a few months prior to my arrival at the compound in Seoul in the autumn of 1964.

After interrogating communist espionage agents for six months and being subjected to the knowledge that the prisoners were executed within hours of the termination of my interrogation, one of my fellow interrogators confided in me that the officers had been watching me closely for signs that I might break under the daily stress of the job. I am proud that I stayed the course, although my ulcers had not disappeared nearly two years following my discharge.

The facts of the situation, including the timeline of events beginning with the bold, bloodless coup by General Chung Hee Park (Park Chung Hee) on May 16, 1961 and ending on November 4, 1965, the day I took my final glimpse of Seoul as the passenger plane lifted off, banked to the left in a wide arc, leveled off and appeared to remain suspended in the sky before choosing to head in the direction of California and home, paint a four-year picture of an economically poor country attempting desperately to gain purchase and move into the modern world, while being thwarted at every turn by communist North Korea.

I was able to not only *observe* life in both South Korea and North Korea during this period of painful upheaval on the Korean peninsula, but to actually play an active role in these national affairs as a member of the elite seven-man prisoner interrogation team at the vaunted 502nd Military Intelligence Battalion.

Within a few months of my arrival at the 502, straight from the U.S. Army Intelligence Center in Baltimore, Maryland, and eager to put my prisoner interrogation skills to the test, I realized I had joined a unique fraternity of principled, like-minded professionals who placed their duty above all else.

This memoir has included my time spent interrogating only my first six North Korean espionage agents. Of course there were many more interrogations, several of which were followed by midnight one-way rides to the Wall at Inchon inside an enclosed paddy wagon.

However I believe you get the idea. This memoir was never intended to be a detailed compendium of the North Korean espionage agents whom I interrogated, nor a running commentary on the mutual hatred and ill will of brothers facing brothers across the DMZ. Rather this work is a true account of four years, four months and four days in the life of a young man held in awe and wonderment over a situation he never could have envisioned and would not have believed if his adventure had been lived by someone else.

Closing Thoughts and Lessons Learned

Upon reflection many years after living my life as the sole feature writer for the *Stars & Stripes* daily newspaper and following that as a Prisoner of War interrogator, I was convinced I had been occupying a front-row seat in one of Swift's surrealistic Lilliputian adventures.

And during this time I sometimes wondered – but never voiced aloud of course – when I would be found out; when the U.S. Army brass would determine that my reporting on all those more than a dozen meetings of the Military Armistice Commission (MAC) was not up to a journalist's professional standards.

Likewise for my interrogation and analysis of North Korean communist spies' plans to once again invade South Korea. Because somewhere along the line I had come to question whether my responsibilities had overwhelmed me, that an older, more experienced, more intelligent person could have done a better job. Self-doubt can be terminal even when taken in small doses.

However following an extended period of self-analysis, fortunately I came to a conclusion most favorable to my long-term mental well-being, and I stored forever out of sight any nagging doubts I may have entertained during the period in question.

In my defense I am proud to report that during my fifteen months as the feature writer for the *Stars & Stripes*, I never once received a negative critique of my writing nor had my facts questioned.

During these fifteen months I drove to Panmunjom to listen to and observe fourteen meetings of the Military Armistice Commission (MAC), and my analysis of the proceedings was the closest anyone came to an official account of those meetings. I have always been proud of the trust placed in me by Col. Creel and Bureau Chief Sergeant Warren Kelsey.

The astute Eighth U.S. Army physician had impressed upon me the need to make a clean break with my army past upon the end of my tour with the 502, in order to leave my ulcers and the cause of said ulcers in my past, which he said is where they belonged. I agreed with the physician.

My final decision not to re-enlist centered on the mental and emotional fatigue caused by the nature of the mission. I had developed a full-blown case of the ulcers and the physicians at Eighth U.S. Army headquarters had several times suggested that I transfer out of the 502. However my devotion to duty had precluded me from taking this route. What the 502 colonel had said was true – the U.S. Army, *at my request*, had expended a great deal of time and resources into making me a prisoner interrogator, and I could not renege on my part of the bargain yet remain true to my core values.

Post Traumatic Stress Disorder? What Else But?

And each day that passed, moving me another day closer to my departure date, served to confirm that indeed my decision had been a sound one. In the interest of completing the record, I will briefly enumerate the reasons that supported my decision, though not necessarily in any particular order of importance.

I saw the writing on the wall the night the South Korean Army M.P. guards drove up to the far corner of the compound and loaded my *second* prisoner into the oversized paddy wagon for the final ride to his execution.

At that time I had been falling asleep nightly for longer than two months, recalling the screams of my *first* prisoner as he had been driven to his end.

Now suddenly I had *two* communist espionage agents to ensure that from that night forward I never would enjoy a full night's sleep as long as I remained at the 502.

There is definitely a downside to being possessed with a vivid imagination. And the best characterization of this phenomenon as far as I was concerned came in the form of flashbacks of the image my mind conjured up pertaining to the execution of doomed communist espionage agents just off the two-lane Seoul-Inchon road in the wee hours of the morning, just a few hours after I signed the Final Interrogation Summary, effectively concluding the interrogation that had delayed the prisoner's execution for several months.

Thus if I re-enlisted for another tour at the 502, I would be forced to revisit this same trauma on a daily basis, compounding the mental anguish that caused my ulcers initially.

Add to this the constant pressure to produce results that had hatched my ulcers after only four months at the 502, and there was again no way for this situation to improve. We seven dedicated prisoner interrogators needed professional counseling on a regular basis. However Post Traumatic Stress Disorder (PTSD) was not even recognized by the U.S. Army in 1964-65. At least not at the 502.

The physician's admonition did not fall on the proverbial "deaf ears." As far as this is concerned the fears centering around my health alone could have justified my decision. However there were several contributing factors worthy of mention here.

One of the factors in my decision to call it quits and return to my civilian life was the fact that from the beginning I never had any intention of making the army a career. Had this been the case I would have signed up for Officer Candidate School (OCS) when I first enlisted in the army after graduation from college in May 1961. I had selected the Army simply because enlistment was for three years whereas enlistment in the Navy, Air Force and Marines was for four years.

Korea, prisoner interrogation and writing for the *Stars & Stripes* were adventures that I embarked upon simply because the opportunities and challenges presented themselves, yet still left me many years to continue the pursuit of my established goals – the study of Law, the study of Optometry and beginning my career as a novelist.

Ample evidence that I achieved each of these stated goals is as follows:

On November 4, 1965 I received an Honorable Discharge from the U.S. Army. In September 1967 I enrolled in the University of Houston College of Optometry. In May 1972 I graduated, earning the degree of O.D. (Doctor of Optometry). I have practiced Optometry in Georgia and Florida since 1972.

In September 1977, while practicing Optometry in Ft. Lauderdale, Florida, I was accepted in the Nova Southeastern University College of Law. I graduated in May 1980 with a Juris Doctor (J.D.) degree. I passed the Georgia Bar Exam in February 1980 and the Florida Bar Exam in July 1980. I have been licensed to practice Law in Georgia and Florida since 1980, and have practiced Law in both states.

My career as a novelist is still a work in progress. I began my writing career in 2003. My first book, a memoir entitled *Reflections in an Orphan's Eye: A Decade at Oxford 1947-1957*, was published in 2005. It was an instant best seller, and for nearly a year remained on the list of the *The Publisher's Top Ten Royalty-earning Books*. As of the publishing of *Memories of Distant Places* I have published a total of seventeen books including fifteen mystery novels and two memoirs. The books are listed on amazon.com and barnesandnoble.com under *A. L. Provost*. Please visit me at www.alprovostbooks.com.

Thinking back over the years, the concept of "family" still might have been the ultimate clincher in this momentous decision as to should I stay or should I go. And some of my fellow G.I.s had great difficulty making this abrupt life's change.

No doubt the army life afforded a sense of security. Just do your job and Uncle Sam will take good care of you. The trick is in finding your niche, and in an M.O.S. (Military Occupational Skill) you feel most comfortable.

However there is definitely a downside to becoming a career soldier, especially if one plans to get married and raise a family. In my four years and four months of active duty I served on a total of *seven* different military bases. One can only imagine the strain on a family caused by a wife and a couple of young children literally living like nomads for twenty years. Changing schools every year or two and finding new friends can be quite traumatic for children, especially the younger ones, who need order and security in this screwy, rapidly-changing world.

It is standard practice in the United States Army for a high-ranking officer to conduct an *exit interview* with every soldier who is mustering out of the army and who the military would like to remain on active duty for an additional tour of duty. Thus I knew the colonel would soon be contacting me for this meeting, as my DD Form 214 would indicate my intention not to re-enlist following my sixteen months at the 502.

The colonel's position was the same one I would have taken had our roles been reversed. Namely that the army had invested time and resources in making me a prisoner interrogator. I was indeed earning a lot with two Propays totaling $600 per month, and upon re-enlisting for another three years I would be promoted from Specialist-5 to Specialist-6. I appreciated the fact that he explained my options in a matter-of-fact manner and did not attempt to make the hard sell.

At that interview I decided not to mention the one thing that disturbed me more than all the rest – the physical mistreatment of the North Korean prisoners.

First of all there was no way that the colonel could *not* have known that such abuses existed. Second, I honestly believed there was nothing he could have done to change the tragic situation. I realized that on the return flight to the states, the seat beside me would likely be occupied by two hundred pounds of guilt.

I believe I sensed it was time to go after I had bade farewell to my sixth prisoner. I had not gotten used to my life as a Prisoner of War interrogator – no, this could never happen – but I had begun to slip into the routine of the job, and my relationship with my interrogation partner Col. Kim, was coasting along smoothly. Very professional, the colonel.

As time passed however, I began to observe some noticeable changes in the persona of several of my fellow interrogators.

And I am certain my fellow interrogators had noticed certain changes in my own demeanor.

Although never could I be accused of being the "life of the party," I admit that I was not as outgoing at six months as I had been at four months. At this point I realized it was time to leave the U.S. Army for good, and made arrangements to effect my departure.

I decided to leave any doubts behind at the Oakland, California Processing Center.

I never once questioned my decision to enlist in the U.S. Army on June 30, 1961.

And by the same token I never once questioned my decision to leave the U.S. Army on November 4, 1965. The experience has been unforgettable.

Maintaining Sanity Under Pressure

If there was one quality that applied to each of the dozen or so prisoner interrogators at the 502, it would be dedication to the job borne of pride.

I say the "dozen or so" interrogators because during the sixteen months I worked at the 502 some would rotate stateside only to be replaced by the "new guys," fresh out of the Defense Language Institute and Ft. Holabird's U.S. Army Intelligence Center, definitely the "cream of the crop" at both schools.

There was absolutely no doubt in my mind but that at least a few times during we interrogators' tour at the 502 we all felt the pressure was overwhelming, that we wanted to call it quits and transfer to the motor pool or the typing section. In point of fact a case of the ulcers, to which we all had succumbed by our fifth month, appeared to be our punishment for being stubborn and hanging on for the entire tour.

However each of us appeared to know where he stood in regards to the ulcers affliction. All G.I.s love the spicy Chinese food served in Korean restaurants throughout the country. And any prisoner interrogator at the 502 who dared to ignore the physician's proscription against eating the spicy delicacy would be immediately reminded of this loss of sanity by sharp pains in his stomache. Korean red peppers would do the trick anytime.

The fact that I was the youngest reporter at the *Stars & Stripes* for fifteen months yet was selected to be the only reporter to be charged with covering the more than a dozen meetings of the Military Armistice

Commission at Panmunjom had nothing to do with my age. It was because I was the reporter more trusted by Col. Creel to attend these meetings between the United Nations representatives and the communist Chinese and North Koreans, and to roam the roads of South Korea and come and go as I pleased. For fifteen months no one ever asked me where I was going or when I was coming back. No one.

The only way I knew to repay Col. Creel and Bureau Chief Warren Kelsey's confidence in me was to discover interesting stories to cover and to be spot-on with my facts. The reporter's only stock in trade really, is his accuracy. If I were not certain of my facts I simply did not write the story. This should be the reporter's Code of Conduct.

Just as my first memoir *Reflections*, was written from the heart, I hope you have enjoyed reading my *Memories of Distant Places* as much as I have enjoyed writing the book.

And now, for the rest of the story…

With my promise to be brief I believe I should bring my adventure up to date. Fortunately I did survive ten long years of incarceration in Oxford Orphanage with my sanity intact. In addition although the army gave me a voucher to use in case I needed to continue treatment of my ulcers following my discharge from the army on November 4, 1965, I harked back to the advice of the army physician at the Yongsan infirmary in Seoul. He stressed my need for a *total* break with the 502.

As I walked out the front door of the Oakland, California Processing Center with my Separation Orders in hand, I observed a large trash container standing about ten feet from the door. Without giving it any conscious thought I tore the voucher into two neat pieces, tossed them into the trash can and continued walking, completing my break with my recent past – the U.S. Army and the infamous 502.

My plan following my discharge was to work toward degrees in Optometry and Law. I applied for admission to the University of Houston College of Optometry. The next class began in September 1967.

While waiting for classes to begin I became a computer systems analyst at Pratt & Whitney at its research and development center (on aircraft engines), located in Palm Beach County, Florida.

In April 1967, to be closer to the University of Houston I ended my employment at Pratt & Whitney Aircraft and took a similar position at NASA outside Houston.

I started classes in September 1967. I also became the night shift supervisor in Building 12, the main computing complex located adjacent to the Mission Control Building at NASA.

Between September 1967 and May 1972 I attended classes at the University of Houston College of Optometry during the day, and worked as the Building 12 supervisor at night. If an astronaut went to the moon between September 1967 and June 1972, I knew him and interacted with him on a regular basis. The best adjective I would choose to describe these professionals is *dedicated*.

Following graduation from Optometry School in May 1972, my wife and two children, Derek and Karen, moved to Ft. Lauderdale, Florida, where I opened my Optometry office.

In 1977 I started classes at Nova Southeastern University College of Law, located in Ft. Lauderdale. I graduated in May 1980. I passed the Georgia Bar exam in February 1980 and the Florida Bar exam in July 1980. I have practiced Law and Optometry in Georgia and Florida for forty years.

My wife Evelyn is also an attorney, licensed to practice Law in Georgia and Florida. We have been married since 1967. The last time we counted we have four grown children, eight grandchildren and four great-grandchildren.

More Recognition

I graduated from Berry College in 1961. Nearly a half century later, in November, 2009, I received a letter from Clara McRae, Vice President, Association Awards, Berry Alumni Association. The letter follows:

November 13, 2009

Dear Alton:

Congratulations! You have been nominated for the Berry Alumni Association's *Distinguished Achievement Award*. The recipient of this award will show evidence of the following criteria:

III. The recipient has achieved success above average.

IV. The recipient has achieved leadership/success within the local level.

V. The recipient has achieved recognition/honors within her/his occupation or professional field.

VI. The recipient has achieved outstanding leadership within a significant organization above the local level.

Using the above criteria, the Association's awards committee will select the three top nominees for this award and submit their applications to a committee of business and professional people who have no connection with Berry. This committee of professionals will make the final, unbiased selection.

Award winners will be notified in April 2010. Awards will be presented during Alumni Weekend on Friday,

May 21, 2010. Distinguished alumni award winners have their names entered into the Alumni Hall of Fame in Berry's Alumni Center.

Again, congratulations! Your nomination for this award is an honor. Please complete the enclosed application and return it to the Office of Alumni Relations by December 15, 2009. You may also complete the form online by going to www.berry.edu/alumni. Access the form by clicking on the link in the block on the right. Please choose the form for Distinguished Achievement.

Sincerely,
Clara H. McRae
Vice President, Association Awards
Berry Alumni Association

With a confused heart, I felt compelled to withdraw my name from the short list of three nominees for consideration. My reasoning follows.

It wasn't that I didn't think I deserved the honor. No, I have always reserved a soft spot in my heart for Martha Berry's ideals.

No, it is just that once I really gave the situation a lot of thought, I simply believed that among all those thousands of Berry alumni, surely there had to be several dozen more deserving than I of this prestigious award.

Closing on a Lighter Note

As mentioned above I worked as a computer systems analyst at NASA while waiting for classes to begin at the University of Houston College of Optometry in the fall of 1967.

Recall that in 1967 *personal computers* had not been invented. The only computers in use were called *mainframe* computers, and when a computer programmer started *running a job* on the IBM 360 or the Univac 1107, for example, the first thing the computer operator – not the same as the computer programmer – did was to feed large metal trays of *punchcards* into the mainframe.

I had begun dating Evelyn Fuentes, a graduate electronics engineer, shortly after mustering out of the army on November 4, 1965. We both worked for Pratt & Whitney Aircraft at its Research and Development Center located in Palm Beach County, Florida.

In order for me to be prepared to enter the University of Houston College of Optometry in early September 1967, Evelyn and I married on March 25, 1967, quit our jobs at Pratt & Whitney Aircraft and accepted employment at Lockheed Electronics Company near the NASA Manned Spacecraft Center in Houston.

On August 15, 1967 I informed my supervisor at Lockheed that I had decided to attend Optometry School full time, beginning on September 7, 1967.

"Are classes held only during the day?" asked my supervisor.

Under the circumstances I thought this to be a strange question. Yet I was always open to opportunities. So I asked her to explain. This explanation follows.

Upon arriving in Texas from Florida in March 1967 my wife and I purchased a home in Clear Lake City (pop. 15,000), situated but a few miles from NASA.

Ninety percent of the work at NASA was performed by contractors, who answered to what were known as *NASA Monitors*. The largest contractor by far was Lockheed Electronics Company, that was wholly-owned by Lockheed Aircraft Company.

The two most important buildings on the NASA grounds were *Mission Control* and the adjacent *Main Computing Complex*, also known as *Building 12*.

In the Mission Control building one could see the technicians sitting at long tables staring at monitors in front of them. These were called *monitors* because they monitored, or tracked, certain activity of the spacecraft in flight. However these television-like instruments were not computers. Rather any *computing*, as the word is commonly used, was done in the adjacent Main Computing Complex (Building 12).

"Coincidentally at this time we are in need of a systems analyst to take over the position as Night Shift Supervisor in the Main Computing Complex," explained my supervisor.

The position came with a substantial increase in salary. I supervised 16-20 employees and coordinated my schedule with the NASA Monitor. I accepted the job offer and we set a date for me to show up at 11:30 p.m. to meet my employees.

Starting Off on the Wrong Foot?

I arrived at the parking lot in front of Mission Control and the Main Computing Complex at around 11:15 p.m. As it was nighttime there were very few cars in the large parking lot. Having my choice of parking spaces, I parked in the very first row, got out of my car and walked the short distance to the Main Computing Complex.

I met the second shift supervisor, who had assembled the third shift employees, and introductions were made all around. I had closed the door to the large office in order to keep out the ambient noise in the hallways.

I had just begun addressing the meeting when suddenly there came the harsh rapping of large knuckles on the door. I stepped to the door and opened it to find filling the space of the opened door, one really godawful huge NASA guard in uniform, with strapped on his bulky hip the largest handgun I had ever seen. Standing behind him and to the side was another one just like him. Both these men could have played first string tackle for the Baltimore Colts.

Before I could utter a greeting or invite them into the office the first one spoke.

"Who is Mr. Provost?"

"I am Mr. Provost. How may I help you?" I managed to squeak out, looking from one security guard to the other, apprehensively.

"Come with us," said the first guard. Since this did not sound like a request, without comment I moved toward the door as the two guards stepped out of my way. The three of us marched down the long hall and out the front door of the Main Computing Complex side-by-side, with myself sandwiched between the two of them. Nobody spoke a word.

Presently we approached four men standing beside my light blue, 2-door 1967 Kharmann Ghia, that was Volkswagen's version of the sports car. The nighttime lighting was poor, so I did not recognize any of the men by sight. However I did note that one of the men was somewhat shorter in stature than the others.

So there we stood in the semi-darkness, the two security guards, the four men standing around my Kharmann Ghia, and I. And one of the seven men still didn't know why he seemed to be the main attraction in this NASA midnight drama.

"Mr. Provost, I would like you to meet Col. Frank Borman," said the first security guard. The shorter of the four men stepped toward me and held out his hand, that I shook while still not knowing the reason why.

"Col. Borman is the Commander of the upcoming Apollo 8 moon flight," added the guard. And up until this moment I still did not have the slightest clue as to why I was there.

"It's so nice to meet you, Col. Borman," I said. "What can I do for you, sir?" I said while surreptitiously wiping my sweaty right palm on my right pants leg.

"You can move your car, Provost," said Col. Borman, laughing with the other three men who were wearing civilian clothes.

The colonel good-naturedly slapped me on the back, adding, "You've stolen my parking place, son."

"I'm so sorry, colonel," I apologized. "I guess I didn't see any signs. I've never parked here in the dark before, and this is my first night on the job as night shift supervisor in the Main Computing Complex."

"It's an understandable mistake," said the colonel as he knelt down in front of the concrete bumper guard in front of my car.

I knelt down also, to where I could see the stenciled *Col. FRANK BORMAN* on the front of the concrete bumper. After apologizing again I shook hands with the colonel, and moved my car to a space about five rows back, making sure the bumper guard did not have anyone's name stenciled on it.

And then I had to walk back inside and explain my colossal blunder to my new night shift crew.

I could never have envisioned a more inauspicious beginning to my new job as Third Shift Supervisor in the Main Computing Complex. However they weren't finished with me just yet.

The main computers in use were the Univac 1106, 1007 and the 1108, that was solely used for NASA's internal computer programs. And the majority of the programs to be run on the 1108 were done on Third Shift. The procedure was somewhat as follows:

When a NASA program was to be run, I would receive a telephone call from the NASA Security Office located in Mission Control. I would literally "drop everything" and walk over to Mission Control, where a security guard would be waiting with the discs to be used on the program. I would sign for the discs, collect them and the armed security guard would escort me back to the Main Computing Complex.

I would give the discs to the Lead Computer Operator (not the programmer) and the guard and I would observe as the Computer Operator fed the discs into the mainframe and initiated the computer program on the 1108.

The end product of running the program was nearly always a paper printout of from 50 to 200 pages. The Lead Computer Operator would box up the input discs and the paper printout, tape the closed box, give the box to me, and the guard and I would return to Mission Control, where a Receiving Security Guard would sign for the materials. I would then return to the Main Computer Complex and continue my night.

The Real Reason Apollo 8 Could Not Land on the Moon

I took much good-natured ribbing about taking Col. Borman's parking space in front of Mission Control. Occasionally we would meet in the parking lot – I coming to work at 11:00 p.m. and he just leaving the parking lot at that time. We would greet one another and the colonel would remind me not to take his parking space. Again.

Before long I had met all the astronauts. They knew me as simply "Provost," and I insisted on addressing each of them by his military rank.

In 1968 Americans were ready to see an American *moon-landing*. But first the Apollo 8 team had to perform a trial flight, in other words fly to the moon, slow down to be trapped as a satellite of the moon, make ten orbits of the moon, and finally return safely to earth.

Crew members selected for this flight were Jim Lovell, Bill Anders and Frank Borman. Col. Borman was named Flight Commander. Liftoff of the rocket occurred on Saturday, December 21, 1968 at 7:51 a.m. With each lunar orbit made, Americans observing back home hoped that this would be the landing.

At about the fifth of the ten orbits one of the employees asked to nobody in particular why had the crew not landed on the moon but continued orbiting it.

"Oh my god, I'll bet Provost has gone and stolen Borman's parking space again," came the quick reply, followed by raucous laughter.

I suppose I'll never live this one down.

Since 1984 I have practiced Optometry (a lot) and Law (not as much) outside Atlanta. In 2003 I began my writing career, that has been successful.

My first book, a memoir entitled *Reflections in an Orphan's Eye* and subtitled *A Decade at Oxford 1947-1957*, was published in 2005. Two months following publication the book had jumped to No. 5 on the publisher's list of *Top Ten Royalty Earning Books* and remained on the coveted list for almost a year. I was honored.

In addition I have written and published 16 mysteries. I have my books critiqued by *Writer's Digest Magazine*, and I am pleased to report that although some reviews are naturally better than others, all the reviews have been good.

I sincerely trust that you have enjoyed reading *Memories of Distant Places*, and if so, wholeheartedly recommend to you *Reflections in an Orphan's Eye: A Decade at Oxford 1947-1957*. Thank you for your interest.

- The End -

www.ingramcontent.com/pod-product-compliance
Lightning Source LLC
LaVergne TN
LVHW091531060526
838200LV00036B/568